The Care and
Management of
NATIVE
PONIES

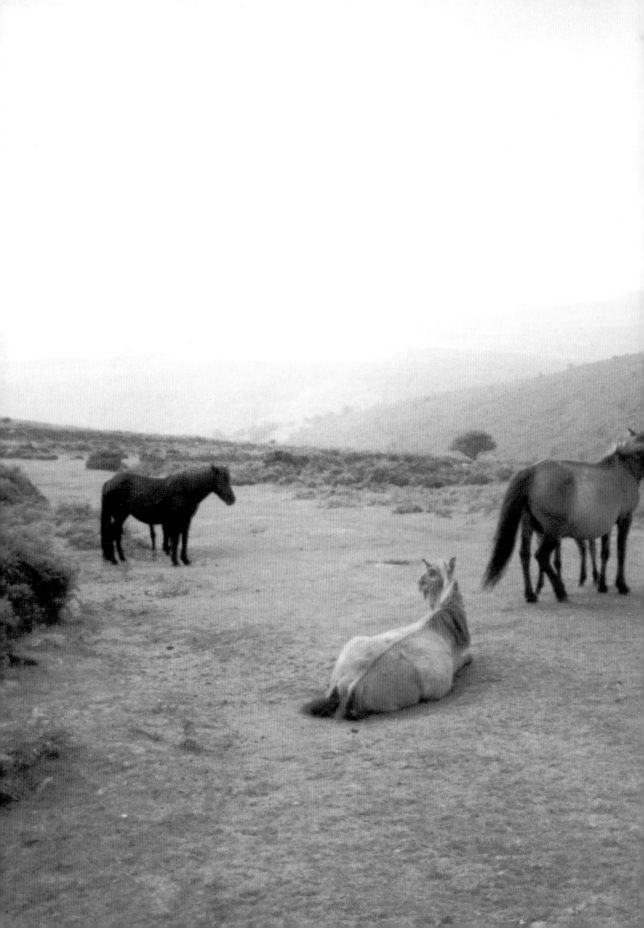

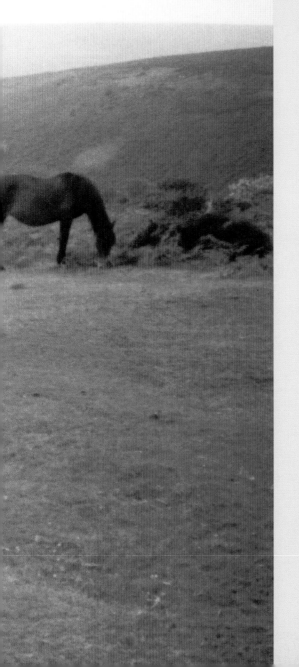

The Care and Management of
NATIVE PONIES

An Owner's Manual

JENNY
MORGAN

J. A. ALLEN

Photograph on previous page:
Wild Dartmoor Ponies

British Library Cataloguing-in-Publication Data.
A catalogue record for this book is available from the
British Library.

ISBN 0.85131.768.5

Published in Great Britain in 2000
by J. A. Allen
an imprint of Robert Hale Ltd.
Clerkenwell House,
45-47 Clerkenwell Green,
London, EC1R 0BT.

Typeset by Textype Typesetters, Cambridge
Colour separation by Tenon & Polert Colour
Scanning Ltd.
Printed by
Kyodo Printing Co (S'pore) Pte Ltd
Illustrations by Julie Williams and Chris Belcher
Diagram on page 122 by Rodney Paull
Designed by Judy Linard

Contents

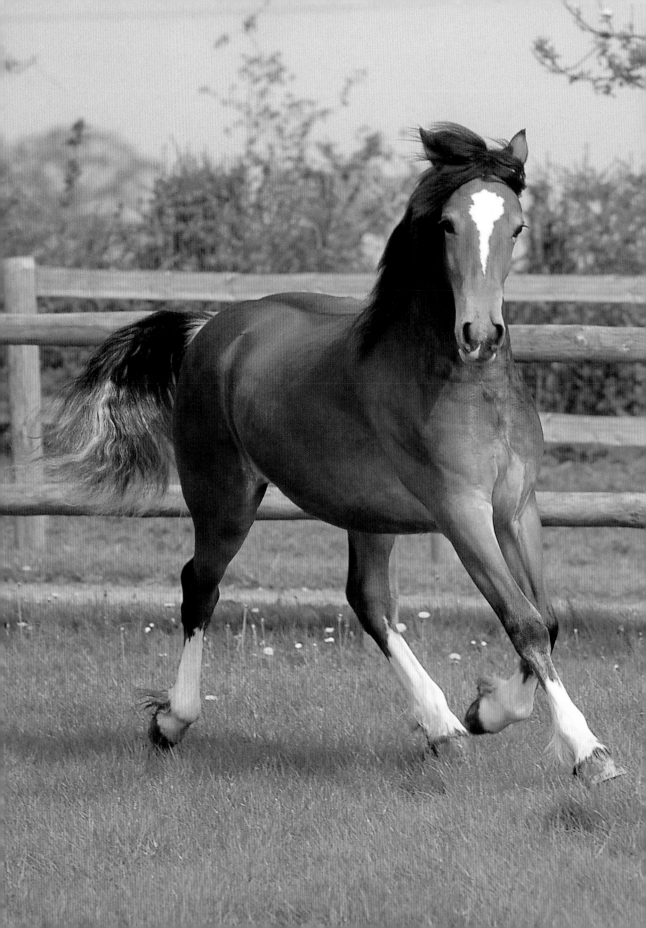

Acknowledgments

Thanks to Caroline Burt of J. A. Allen for giving me the opportunity to write this book and to John Beaton for his patient support. Thanks are also due to those many people who supplied photographs of their lovely ponies.

Grateful thanks are due to the Society of Authors who provided welcome financial support from the Authors Foundation fund, for vital research.

Most of all thanks are due to the many native ponies who have enriched my life over the last forty years. They include my very first Welsh pony, Chieveley Honey known to her friends as Whisky and who sadly went to the big stable in the sky during the writing of this book. Also mentioned must be Whisky's best friend, the well known Aston Tinkerbell, proof, if it were needed, that native ponies are long lived, and my current show campaign team Aston True Welshman and Ballan Blodwen. Every single one of them has given me times of great joy and times of enormous frustration. Anyone who has never owned a native pony has never lived!

The author and publishers are grateful to the following for permission to reproduce copyright photographs in this book : Bob Langrish, title page, pages 13, 15, 16, 18, 20, 23, 24, 26, 28, 29, 31, 33, 50, 67, 83, 101, 104, 112; Mrs J. Eakin, pages 8, 64; Mrs V. James, page 21; Mrs D. Jordan, page 30; Saltire Stables, pages 44, 48; Karen Coumbe, pages 69, 70, 93; Sue Devereux, pages 94, 95; Jane Beaton, pages 97, 98, 127; Mrs R. Abrahall, page 142. All other photographs supplied by Jenny Morgan.

Welsh Section D yearling

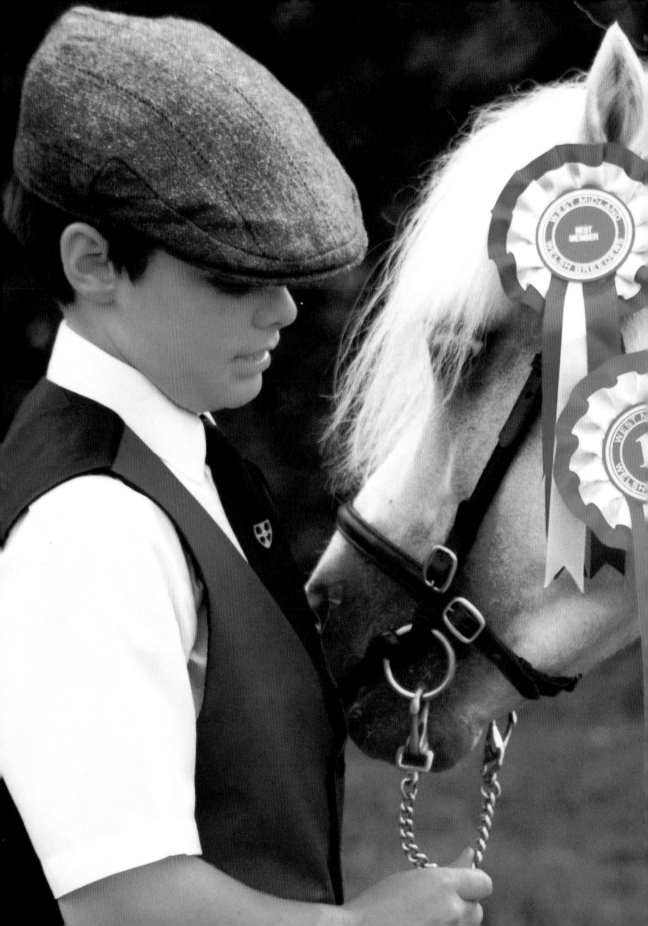

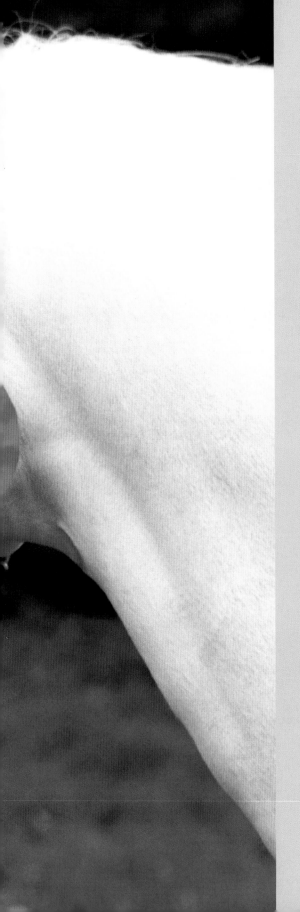

Introduction

Anyone with an interest in horses and ponies knows our native breeds – they are everywhere. At every show and in every Pony Club, riding club and hunt in the country. They have always been around – or have they? In fact our breeds as they are established today are a relatively recent arrangement. Most stud books and breed standards have been around for less than one hundred years. This is not to say that the ponies have not always been there but it is only relatively recently that the breeds have become so very separately defined and documented, and recorded. Whilst ponies have roamed the mountains of Wales since records began, they only became the four sections of the stud book, as they are known today, in this century. Breeders of Welsh Cobs and admirers of stallions kept some records and the pedigrees and achievements of various animals were passed on from generation to generation by word of mouth but the practice of issuing registration papers only began at the beginning of this century. This example is fairly common in all our breeds, with the Shetland stud book being the oldest.

Sammiejoe Eakin with Welsh Section A stallion Vogue Twister

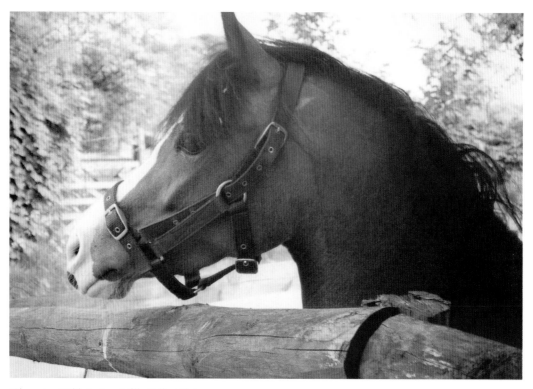

Champion Welsh Section A filly Ballan Blodwen

In the last thirty years or so, the popularity of native ponies has accelerated apace. At a show in the Midlands in 1980 there was only one entry in the National Pony Society ridden mountain and moorland championship qualifier. At the same show in 1998 there were more than twenty entries in each of four sections – an entry approaching a hundred ponies.

This is absolutely typical of show entries in both ridden and in-hand native classes across the country. Whilst there were horse shows in the first half of the century, they had a strong agricultural bias. Now a whole new 'hobby' has grown up around the huge numbers of shows that take place every week, winter and summer, all over the country. The native pony has taken well to

his role in this activity, proving himself a natural showman both in-hand and under saddle. Huge numbers of people, new to keeping horses, can start off with a native pony for relatively little expenditure compared to a thoroughbred hack or hunter but have just as much fun and be just as much part of the show.

However, shows are only part of the life of native ponies. Thousands and thousands of native ponies compete every week across the country in every possible kind of equestrian event. Thousands more are well loved hacks for children and adults, providing a safe and sensible conveyance for those who wish to just view the countryside from the back of a horse. Others are kept as pets. These ponies having finished their ridden or breeding career and being generally long lived make ideal companions for youngsters both equine and human.

With more people having more leisure time, riding is one of the activities which has seen a steady increase in popularity since the war. Hardly any native ponies are kept strictly for work now, unless you count working in a riding school or trekking centre. Working horses on farms or ponies being used for transport are now far less often seen. The native pony has changed well into his role as provider of a mount for 'fun' activities.

What else besides a native pony can live on very little; if properly supervised can live out all year round; can work unshod unless he does much road work; is usually healthy, hardy and easy to keep well? What amazing value for money he is!

This book aims to help the complete beginner to care for their pony properly and sensibly. It also hopes to give useful advice and helpful tips to the more experienced owner. Last but by no means least it comes with the thought that if you have even half as much joy from native ponies as I have had then your life will be greatly enriched.

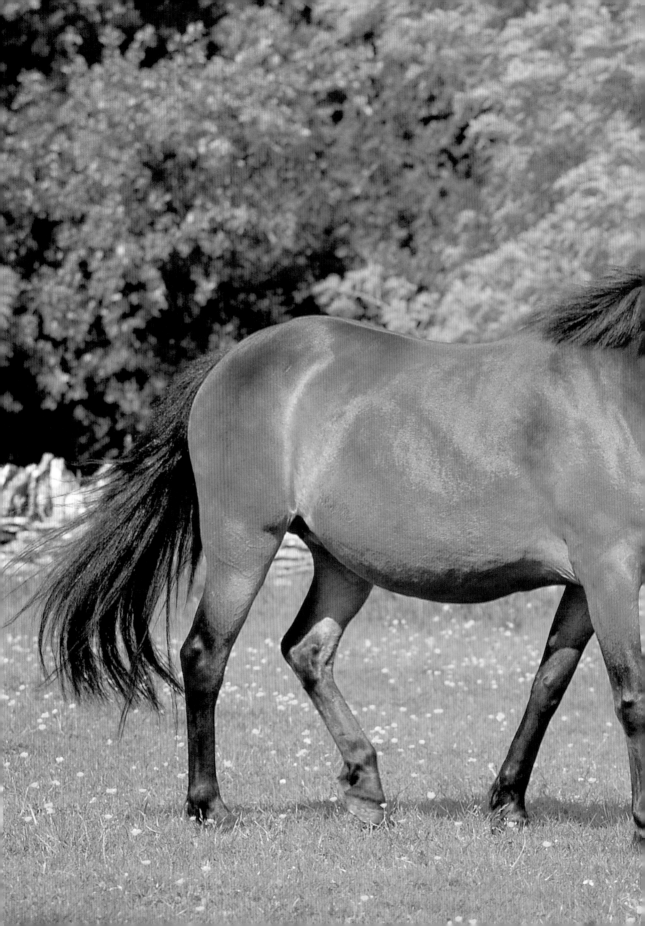

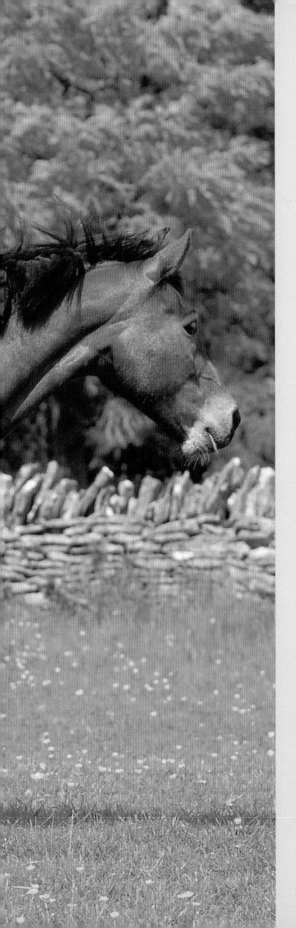

1

History and Origins

All breeds of native ponies have certain aspects in common, such as hardiness and hairiness and all breeds have something very different and distinctive, which is theirs alone. In historical documents, references to horses and ponies, especially detailed references are not common.

However, the native breeds as we know them today were well documented in the twentieth century. Pedigrees can be traced back through stud books and most of the breeds have changed very little in that time. There has been a certain refinement of some breeds to make them more suitable as show animals or for riding, but a Shetland pony, kept in all his life and rugged up will still grow a coat suitable for life on Shetland if he is suddenly thrown in the field one winter. This is the same process which means that dogs which have their tails docked are still born with long tails no matter how many litters are docked.

The breed standards included in this chapter are reproduced as written by the various breed societies. Sometimes the language used is not easy for a novice to understand. However, the societies are there to promote their breed and without exception welcome queries from owners and potential owners of their particular breed. The most important thing to remember is that good conformation is good conformation whatever the breed and generally speaking a pony with good conformation (and most particularly with good limbs) will put less strain on its joints and muscles when it is working and therefore stays sound for longer than one with poor conformation and consequent possible problems. It is a very useful skill to be able to assess conformation and the only way to learn this is by practise.

The Shetland Pony

Shetlands are the smallest of our native breeds and are of the most northern origin. Ponies of a Shetland type can be seen in cave paintings dating from the Stone Age and on the Bressay Stone, a Celtic monument. At Sumburgh an Iron Age site has been excavated and bones of Shetland type ponies, thought to date from a period of between 100BC and AD100 were found. When the eighteenth century priest and traveller the Rev. John Brand visited the Shetland Isles in 1701 he reported: 'They have a sort of little horse called Shelties . . . some will be 9 or 10 Nevis or Handbreadths high . . . They will live till a considerable age as 26, 28 or 30 years, and they will be good riding horses in 24 especially they'll be more vigorous and live longer if they be 4 years old before they are

put to work. Those of a black colour are judged to be the most durable, and the Pyed often proves not so good.'

Nothing has really changed for Shetland enthusiasts, because black Shetlands are still thought by some breeders to be the best. They still live to a ripe old age and they are still durable and hardy.

In around 1820 a Mr Youett reported that 'one of them, nine hands in height, carried a man of 12 stone 40 miles in one day.'

The Shetland Pony stud book was founded in 1890 and first published in 1891. The first recorded pony is number 22 Lion, foaled in 1864, a dun, 36 inches. It appears that at this time the most prominent colours were a 'dark mouse grey' and various duns.

About this time an attempt was made to increase the size of the breed with larger ponies being brought from Norway. A distinct breed, being a Shetland cross and called the Sumburgh was established. However, pure Shetlands were still very much the majority of the population and the blood can be taken to be pure for well over a hundred years and possibly for two thousand!

Shetland Ponies can be any colour except spotted and recently skewbald has been somewhat in fashion – as indeed it is in general 'pony' fashion. However, it should be said here that none of the other native breeds allow piebald and skewbald. The Shetland Pony has a wonderful double coat in the winter which has longer guard hairs which allow the water to run off and not soak the softer insulating under coat. It is now permissible to clip the coat of

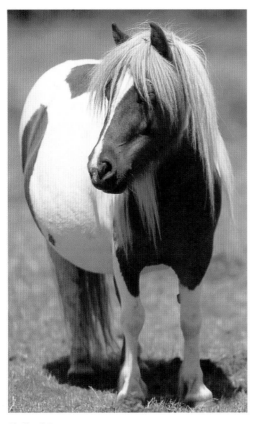

Shetland Pony

stars in the Shetland Pony Grand National at Olympia. Often shown on television when excerpts from the show are seen in amongst the show jumping, his courage, jumping ability and amazing speed for his size are all apparent.

BREED STANDARD

Height: Registered stock must not exceed 40in (102cm) at two years or under, or 42in (107cm) at four years or over. Ponies are measured from the withers to the ground with a measuring stick, and a level stance, preferably concrete, should be used.

Colour: Shetland ponies may be any colour except spotted.

Coat: The coat changes according to the seasons of the year. A double coat in winter with guard hairs which shed the rain and keep the pony's skin completely dry in the worst of the weather but in contrast, the summer coat is short and should carry a beautiful silky sheen. At all times, the mane and tail hair should be long, straight and profuse, the feathering of the fetlocks straight and silky.

Head: The head should be small, carried well, and in proportion. Ears should be small and erect, wide-set, but pointing well forward. Forehead should be broad with bold, dark, intelligent eyes. Blue eyes are not acceptable. Muzzle must be broad with nostrils wide and open. Teeth and jaw must be correct.

Forelegs: Should be well placed, with sufficient good flat bone. Strong forearm. Short, balanced cannon bone. Springy pasterns.

Hind legs: The thighs should be strong and muscular, with well shaped, strong hocks,

ridden or driven Shetlands during the winter and really it is the only fair way to keep the pony if he is going to be doing any serious work.

Shetlands are very good children's ponies but when buying one you should remember that they have a very big brain for the size of the pony and this can sometimes get them into trouble. Manage a Shetland with this in mind, take no nonsense from him and he will be a friendly and willing companion for any child. Apart from making a success of all children's activities, he drives well and can be used for light farm duties. The Shetland really becomes a household name when he

15

neither hooky nor too straight. When viewed from behind, the hind legs should not be set too widely apart, nor should the hocks turn in.

Feet: Tough, well shaped and round – not short, narrow, contracted or thin.

Action: Straight free action, using every joint and tracking up well.

General: A most salient and essential feature of the Shetland Pony is its general air and vitality (presence), its stamina and its robustness.

The Connemara

The Connemara hails from the west of Ireland and has long been the partner in work and play of the indigenous people of the Connemara region. He is often pictured carrying seaweed for fertiliser and turf for fuel. The origins of the breed are not known for sure but merchants in the area traded with Spain, so there was almost certainly an element of Arab or Barb blood. This is seen in the elegance of the pony today.

Founded in 1923, the breed society has done much to improve and conserve the breed. The English Connemara Pony Society, founded less than 50 years ago – and thus the

Connemara Ponies

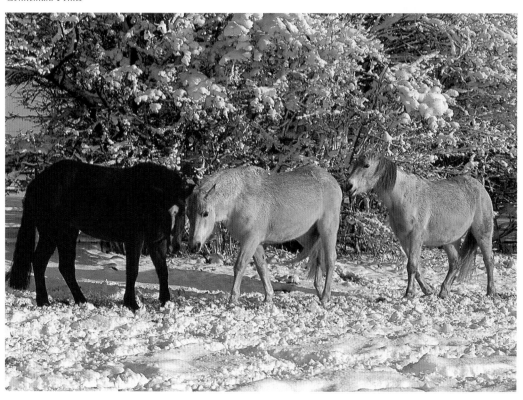

youngest of the native breed societies –
has carried on the valuable work. The
pony today is up to 148 cm (just over
14.2hh) and therefore provides a good
ride for a smaller adult. Indeed many
Connemaras have found fame in
competition being junior eventers and
dressage ponies as well as ridden and
working hunter ponies. Part bred
Connemaras compete in every sphere of
equitation. The Connemara provides a
large native to cross with a Thoroughbred
and the result makes an excellent
competition horse of a good size.

Many Connemaras are ridden ponies
and therefore clipped during the winter but
nevertheless the native blood is still there
and a Connemara could easily winter out if
necessary.

An intelligent pony and a renowned
jumper, the Connemara is a very good
second pony or teenager's ride. They can
very often be of sufficient quality to
compete under British Show Pony Society
(B.S.P.S.) rules in working and show hunter
pony classes. This means that they have two
sets of classes in which to compete – two
bites of the cherry!

BREED STANDARD

Characteristics: Excellent temperament;
hardiness and staying power; intelligence
and soundness; surefootedness and jumping
ability; suitable for a child or adult.

Height: 52–58in (133–148cm).

Colour: Grey, bay, black, brown, and dun
with occasional roan, chestnut, palomino,
and dark-eyed cream.

Type: Compact, well balanced riding type
with depth, substance and good heart-
room, standing on short legs covering a lot
of ground.

Head: Well-balanced pony head with
medium length, with good width between
large, dark, kindly eyes. Pony ears, well-
defined cheekbones; jaw relatively deep but
not coarse.

Front: Head set well onto neck. Chest not
overloaded and neck not set on too low.
Well-defined wither and good sloping
shoulder giving a good length of rein.

Body: Deep with strong back. Some length
permissible but should be well ribbed up
with strong loins.

Limbs: Good length and strength in
forearm, well-defined knees and short
cannons with flat bone measuring 7-8in
(18–21cm). Elbows should be free, pasterns
of medium length, feet well shaped of
medium size, hard and level.

Hindquarters: Strong and muscular with
some length, well-developed second thigh
and strong, low set hocks.

Movement: Free and true without undue
knee action, but active and covering the
ground.

The Highland Pony

The headline on the Highland Pony breed
society leaflet says that 'You can take a
Highland anywhere' and when you know
his equable temperament and hardiness
then you can see why this claim is made.
Bred to survive in the worst conditions on
very little food and yet to work hard in
hilly conditions the Highland is a dour
survivor.

Highland Ponies have been mentioned

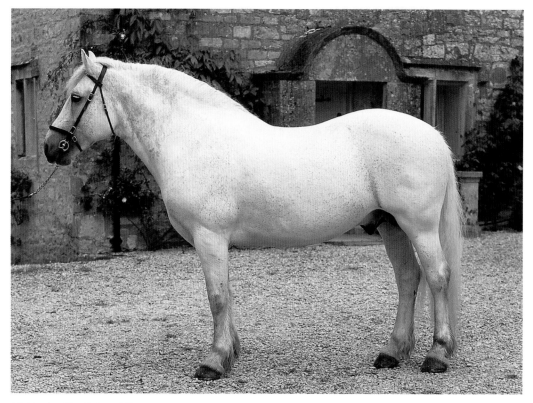

Highland stallion Balmoral Dee

in literature as far back as the 1780s and some pedigrees date back to the 1880s. However, the society of today was started in 1923. It is well known that our present Queen keeps a Highland Stud and that the ponies are used as they have been for many years to bring home shot deer.

The Highland makes a very good choice for a family pony. His steady temperament means that relatively small riders can ride him but he can also carry a heavy man too. Highlands compete in all activities but do excel as driving ponies and for riding long distances in trekking or in competitive long distance riding. Being long lived and cheap to keep, a Highland is ideal for the older owner who will not want to have to change their pony too often.

If you intend to ride your Highland Pony in downland Britain you will probably need to clip him in the winter. His natural thick coat will be more than likely grey or dun, meaning that he will not be so easy to keep clean. However, Highlands do come in other colours, including occasionally bay and liver chestnut – it is just that the majority are light coloured. The long silky flowing mane and tail can prove difficult to deal with. Highland manes and martingales are a tricky combination, however, the flies in the summer are much less bother when you have a full head of hair!

BREED STANDARD

Height: 13hh to 14.2hh.

Mane and tail: Hair should be long, silky and flowing, not coarse. Tail set fairly high and carried gaily.

Colours: Various shades of dun: mouse, yellow, grey, cream, fox. Also grey, brown-black and occasionally bay and liver chestnut with silver mane and tail. Many ponies carry the dorsal eel stripe and many have zebra markings on their forelegs. Apart from a small star, white markings (blazes, socks etc) are disliked and discouraged.

Stallions with white markings, other than a small star, are not eligible for registration.

Head: Well carried, broad between alert and kindly eyes; short between eyes and muzzle, muzzle not pinched, nostrils wide.

Front: Neck strong, not short; good arched top line; throat clean and not fleshy. Shoulders should be well sloped. Withers pronounced.

Body: Compact; back with slight natural curve; chest deep; ribs well sprung.

Quarters: Powerful and strong; well developed thigh and second thigh.

Legs: Flat, hard bone; forearm strong, knee broad; short cannon, pasterns oblique, not too short, well shaped, hard dark hooves. Forearm placed well under the weight of the body; hocks clean and flat. Feather silky and not over-heavy, ending in a prominent tuft at the fetlock.

New Forest

The New Forest Pony dates back to the mists of time. A pot, with a decoration showing a pony and thought to date back to AD300 has been found in the Forest. Much has been done by the Society for the Improvement of New Forest Ponies to sort out a type and to keep up standards for the breed. With a height limit of 14.2hh and ponies seldom being under 12hh the New Forest makes a good teenager's pony or a pony for a larger child. With improvements in breeding, New Forests are appearing that are 'pretty' enough to win B.S.P.S. working or show hunter classes, yet still be a pure native — and have these classes to compete in as well.

Most New Forests seem to be clipped and have pulled manes and tails and indeed you see them winning native classes in this state. The best way to keep them might be to compromise, leaving their mane quite long but having big plaits in classes which require plaited trim.

BREED STANDARD

Height: The upper height limit is 14.2hh. There is no lower limit but ponies are seldom under 12hh.

Colour: New Forest Ponies may be any colour except piebald, skewbald or cream with blue eyes. Bays and browns predominate. White markings on head and legs are permitted. Dark eyed pale palominos and very light chestnuts are only allowed in mares and geldings.

Type: The New Forest Pony should be a riding type with substance. It should have a pony head, well set on, long sloping shoulders, strong quarters, plenty of bone, good depth of body, straight limbs and good hard round feet.

The larger ponies, although narrow

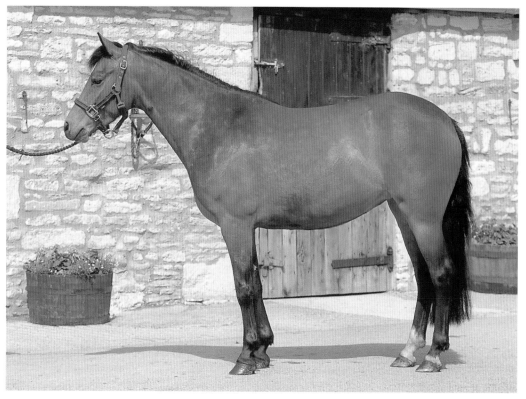

New Forest Pony Peveril Pandora

enough for children are capable of carrying adults. The smaller ponies often show more quality. Judges are requested to give preference to ponies with depth and bone, even at the expense of quality.

Action: Straight, with free movement, but not exaggerated with flicking toes. Over-refined heads are neither typical nor desirable.

The Dales Pony

The Dales Pony was originally bred for the Pennine lead industry and is famous for his weight carrying ability and endurance. They make an excellent harness pony. The stud book when it opened in 1898 made the Dales and Fell out to be two types of the same pony and indeed at that time the two breeds were often crossed. However, with only four registered Dales ponies left in 1955 a separate Dales society was set up in 1963 and the breed goes from strength to strength today.

The height limit is 14.2hh but with the strength and strong trot of this pony their rider needs to be a teenager at least. They are ideal for an adult who wants to ride but not keep a thoroughbred. A Dales Pony can live out all year round and will be cheap and easy to keep. His mane and tail will be naturally long but can be carefully pulled a little if you do not intend to show him and if you find that you keep getting his hair tangled up with your reins. His feather makes him what he is, so do leave it on. It will not be as difficult to look after as you think.

BREED STANDARD

Characteristics: Tremendous stamina; iron constitution; high courage and great intelligence; also calm temperament and very surefooted.

Height: Up to 14.2hh.

Colour: Predominately black with some brown, grey and bay; rarely roan.

Type: Excellent harness ponies, having been used for trotting and for all farm work; the trot is an all-important pace. Famous for their weight carrying abilities and their endurance.

Head: Neat, showing no dish and broad between the eyes. Muzzle relatively small, no coarseness about the jaw and throat, and incurving pony ears. A long forelock, mane and tail of straight hair.

Front: The muscular neck of ample length for a bold outlook, should be set into well-laid sloping shoulders. Short, well-developed forearms set square into a broad chest. Withers not too fine. Stallions should carry a well-arched crest.

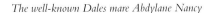

The well-known Dales mare Abdylane Nancy

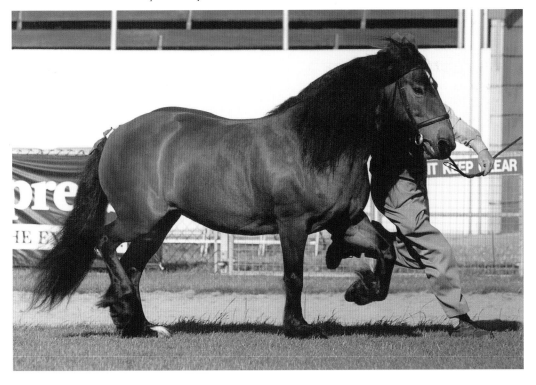

Body: Short-coupled, with strong loins and well-sprung ribs.

Limbs: Cannons, should display an average of 8–9in (20 – 23cm) of flat, flinty bone, with well-defined tendons. Pasterns should be of good length with flexible joints, the hooves large, round and open at the heels with well-defined frogs, and with ample silky, straight feather. Dales are renowned for the quality of their hard, well-shaped feet and legs with beautiful, flat dense bone.

Hindquarters: Lengthy and powerful with very muscular second thighs, above clean, broad flat hocks, well let down.

Movement: Their action is straight and true, they are good movers, really using their knees and hocks for powerful drive. They are renowned for their good trot.

The Fell Pony

Much of what has been said about the Dales Pony applies to the Fell, although the height limit is 14hh. The Fell Pony has characteristic blue feet with extremely strong horn. This means that for an adult who only wants to go for a hack at weekends a Fell Pony would probably not need shoeing.

BREED STANDARD

Height: Not exceeding 14hh.

Colour: Black, brown, bay or grey, preferably with no white markings, though a star or a little white on the hind feet is allowed.

Mane, tail and feathers: Plenty of fine hair (coarse hair is objectionable). All the fine hair, except at the points of the heels may be cast in the summer. Mane and tail are left to grow long.

Head: Small, well chiselled in outline, well set on, forehead broad, tapering to the nose. Nostrils: large and expanding; the eyes prominent, bright, mild and intelligent. Ears: neatly set, well formed and small. Throat and jaws: fine, showing no sign of throatiness or coarseness.

Neck: Of proportionate length, giving good length of rein, strong and not too heavy. Moderate crest in the case of a stallion.

Shoulders: Most important, well laid back and sloping, not too fine at the withers, not loaded at the points, a good long shoulder blade, muscles well developed.

Body: Good strong back, of good outline; muscular loins; deep carcass, and thick through heart; rounded ribcage (from shoulders to flank); short and well coupled. Hindquarters square and strong with tail well set on.

Feet, legs and joints: Feet of good size, round and well formed, open at the heels with characteristic blue horn; fair sloping pasterns, not too long.

Forelegs: Should be straight, well placed and not tied in at the elbows. Big, well formed knees, short cannon bone, plenty of good flat bone below the knee (at least 8in–20cm). Great muscularity of arm.

Hind legs: Good thighs and second thighs, very muscular; hocks well let down and clean cut, plenty of bone below joint – should not be sickle- or cow-hocked.

Action: Walk, smart and true. Trot, well balanced all round with good knee and hock action, going well from the shoulder and flexing the hocks; not going wide or near behind. Should show great pace and

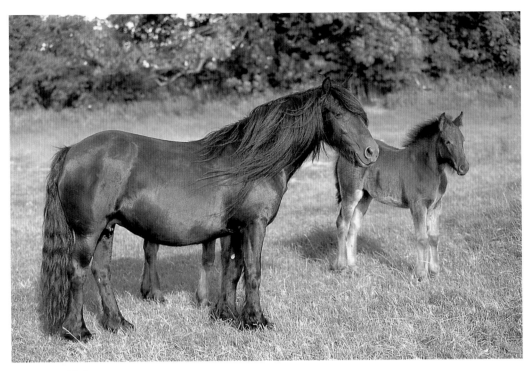

Fell mare and foals

endurance, bringing the hind legs well under the body when going.

General character. Constitutionally the Fell Pony should be as hard as iron; it should show good pony characteristics with the unmistakable appearance of hardiness peculiar to mountain ponies. It should have a lively and alert appearance, and great bone.

The Dartmoor Pony

As the name suggests this breed hails from Dartmoor in the south of England. This moor is a bleak inhospitable place in winter, but moor-bred ponies still survive there today. Being up to 12.2hh in height they are just right for a children's pony though may be too big for some lead-rein and first ridden classes if up to height. The Dartmoor is a very bright character, full of life and always ready for mischief. They can squeeze through the smallest gap in the hedge but only so that they can chat to the ponies next door!

With this good brain, the Dartmoor is usually easy to train and enjoys jumping. Their equable temperament and usual good humour makes a Dartmoor a real companion for a child.

The natural coat is very thick and greasy for life on a wet moor but can be clipped for winter riding. The mane and tail are often long and free flowing but a little careful shortening will not come amiss on a ridden pony. Dartmoor ponies often have very good hooves and for this reason may well be happy working unshod. As with all small natives the tendency to laminitis is one which should be borne in mind.

BREED STANDARD

Height: Not exceeding 12.2hh.

Colour: Bay, brown, black, grey, chestnut, roan. Piebalds and skewbalds are not allowed. Excessive white marking is discouraged.

Head: Should be small, well-set on and (Thoroughbred) blood like, with the nostrils large and expanding, the eyes bright, intelligent and prominent. The ears should be small, well formed, alert and neatly set. The throat and jaws should be fine and showing no sign of coarseness or throatiness.

Neck: Strong, but not too heavy and of medium length. Stallions should have a moderate crest.

Shoulders: Good shoulders are most important. They should be well laid back and sloping, but not too fine at the withers.

Body: Of medium length and strong; well ribbed up and with a good depth of girth, giving plenty of heart room.

Dartmoor Pony Pindox Bracken

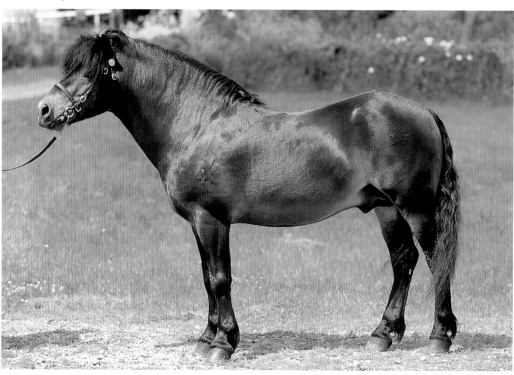

Loin and hindquarters: Strong and well covered with muscle. The hindquarters should be of medium length and neither level nor steeply sloping. The tail is well set up.

Hind legs: The hocks should be well set down with plenty of length from hip to hock, clean cut with plenty of bone below the joint. They should not be sickle- or cow-hocked.

Forelegs: Should not be tied in at the elbows. The forearm should be muscular, and the knee fairly large and flat to the front. The cannon should be short with ample good, flat, flinty bone. The pasterns should be sloping but not too long. The feet should be sound, tough and well shaped.

Movement: Low, straight and free flowing, yet without exaggeration.

General: The mane and tail should be free and flowing. The Dartmoor is a good-looking riding pony, sturdily built yet with quality. In appearance and movement he might be compared to a scaled down version of a middleweight hunter.

The Exmoor Pony

Another bleak moorland inhabitant in the wild and now an officially listed endangered species. For this reason Exmoor Ponies are far less often seen for sale. A pure bred Exmoor will always have a brand showing which herd he belongs to and his herd number. A strong individual, often with a rather stubborn temperament they are not the first choice as a child's pony, despite having a 12.2hh (mares) or 12.3hh (males)

height limit. However, there are exceptions to this and one or two very nice and very well schooled Exmoor ponies have appeared in recent years in ridden classes.

There is not much you can do with an Exmoor coat. It is very hard and dense to protect him from the weather – his own natural New Zealand rug. He is better living out as naturally as possible and should never be clipped or trimmed in any way if he is to be shown.

BREED STANDARD

Height: Stallions and geldings, not exceeding 12.3hh. Mares not exceeding 12.2hh (at any age).

Coat: Close, hard and bright in the summer. Dense and thick in the summer.

Colour: Bay, brown or dun with black points; mealy colour on muzzle, round eyes and inside flanks; no white markings anywhere.

Type: Definite 'pony' character; hard and strong; vigorous and alert; symmetrical in appearance; mealy muzzle and 'toad' eye.

Head and neck: Ears short, thick and pointed; clean cut face; wide forehead; large eyes, wide apart and prominent (toad eye); wide nostrils; mealy muzzle; clean throat; good length of rein.

Shoulders: Clean, fine at the top, well laid back.

Chest: Deep and wide, between and behind the forelegs. Ribs long, deep, well sprung and wide apart.

Back: Level, broad and level across the loins; tail set neatly in.

Legs: Clean and short, with neat, hard feet; forelegs straight, well apart and squarely set; hind legs well apart, neatly perpendicular

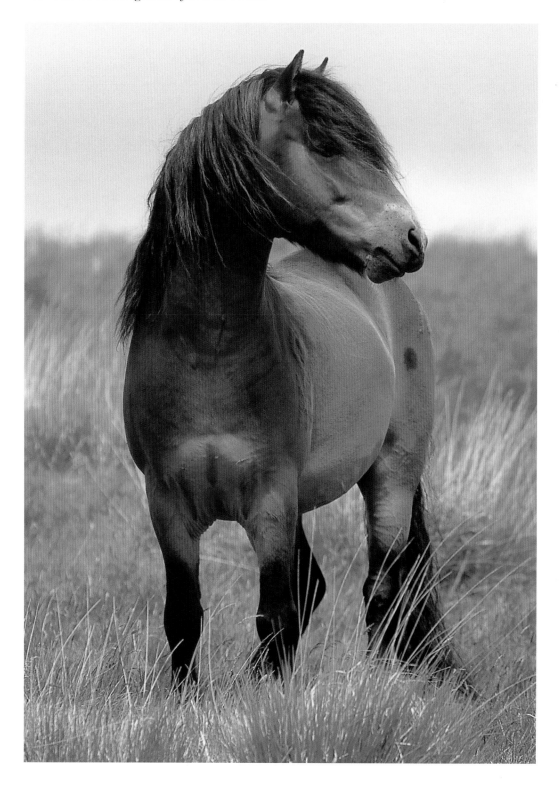

from hock to fetlock, with point of hock in line with the pelvis bone; wide curve from flank to hock joint; legs free in motion with no tendency to sweep or turn.

Action: Straight and smooth, without exaggeration.

Quality: Alert expression with general poise indicating balance and symmetry of movement. Fine clean bone.

Welsh Ponies and Cobs

How clever of the Welsh Pony and Cob Society to evolve a stud book with four sections one of which will give us a pony for every job! Welsh Ponies were originally registered in other stud books such as the Polo Pony Stud Book, but started their own in 1901. The Sections were slightly different then, but with an increase in need for children's riding ponies between the Wars the Section B description was changed and new blood from Arab and Thoroughbred stallions temporarily brought in to accommodate this demand.

SECTIONS A AND B

This is the Welsh Mountain Pony up to 12hh and the Welsh Pony up to 13.2hh. The main difference being the greater height limit for the Section B and as already mentioned the influx of other blood to change this section. Today both sections are still best known as children's ponies. Indeed if you look at the lead-rein and first ridden classes at any show the

Exmoor Pony

majority of ponies will be Welsh Section A with some Section B ponies. It is claimed that Julius Caesar had a stud of Welsh Ponies in North Wales and it is true to say that harness has been found in that area which dates back to Roman times and would have fitted a small Section A.

Welsh Section A and B ponies do anything and everything – Pony Club, hunting, jumping and anything else that is going on. They generally provide a safe conveyance for a child, but can sometimes still show flashes of Welsh fire and this is what gives them great presence.

Many a Welsh Pony has become an institution in a certain area or Pony Club, going from home to home as children outgrow him and with always a new home waiting in the wings and several more lined up behind. They will often live well into their twenties and sometimes thirties, some giving active service for all that time.

Welsh Ponies are very happy living in or out but will probably need clipping for active work in the winter. They tend to shed their coats reasonably early in the spring and this can be very useful for early shows. They make very flashy driving ponies but will always be first and foremost a child's pony. The biggest problem with a Welsh Pony as with all the small natives is the risk of laminitis. This should be borne in mind when making accommodation arrangements.

SECTIONS C AND D

These are the cobs of the Welsh quartet, Section C being the pony of cob type and Section D being the cob. The earliest records of types which resemble today's cobs date from around the sixteenth and seventeenth centuries but even up to the present century cobs were being outcrossed with Hackney and Thoroughbred blood. The stud book was started in 1901.

The Section C pony is increasingly popular today. He can carry a small adult and really enjoys his jumping. He makes a very eye-catching driving pony. Like all the other Welsh Sections he is easy to keep and tough enough to live outdoors.

The Section D is the well-known Welsh cob. He is a true showman – to see the stallions trot up the grand ring at the Royal Welsh show is the best sight in the horse world. He drives, hunts, hacks and jumps with the best of them – a big strong person with stamina and strength. Despite all this fire most cobs are very well mannered and obedient and will not be likely to be nervous of hazards when ridden or driven. Easy to get too fat, they can be kept well on relatively poor grazing such as hill land.

BREED STANDARD
Welsh Mountain – Section A
Height: Not exceeding 12hh.
General character: Hardy, spirited and pony like.

Welsh Mountain Section A - Friars Superted

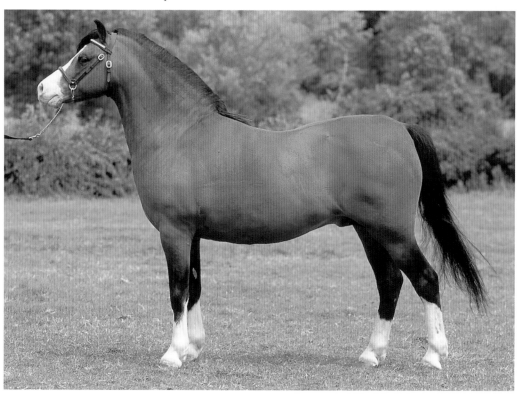

Colour: Any colour, except piebald and skewbald.

Head: Small and clean cut, well set on and tapering to the muzzle. The eyes should be bold and the ears well placed, small and pointed; they should be well up on the head, and proportionately close. The nostrils should be prominent and open. Jaws and throat should be clean and finely cut, with ample room at the angle of the jaw. The silhouette may be concave or 'dished' but never convex or too straight.

Neck: Lengthy, well carried and moderately lean in the case of mares, but inclined to be cresty in the case of mature stallions.

Shoulders: Long and sloping well back. Withers moderately fine but not 'knifey'. The humerus upright so that the foreleg is not set in under the body.

Forelegs: Set square and true, not tied in at the elbows. Long, strong forearm, well developed knee; short flat bone below the knee, pasterns of proportionate slope and length, feet well shaped and round, hooves dense.

Body: Back and loins should be muscular, strong and well coupled. Girth should be deep, the ribs well sprung.

Hindquarters: Lengthy and fine, not cobby, ragged or goose rumped. Tail set on well and carried gaily.

Hind legs: Hocks to be large, flat and clean with points prominent, turning neither inwards nor outwards. The hind leg should not be too bent. The hock set behind a line from the point of the quarter to the fetlock joint. Pasterns of proportionate slope and length. Feet well shaped, hooves dense.

Action: Quick, free and straight from the shoulder, well away in front. Hocks well flexed with straight and powerful leverage, and well under the body.

The Welsh Pony – Section B

Height: Not exceeding 13.2hh.

The general description of the Welsh Mountain Pony can be applied to the Welsh Pony, with greater emphasis being placed on riding pony qualities whilst retaining the true Welsh quality and substance.

Mare and foal - Section B

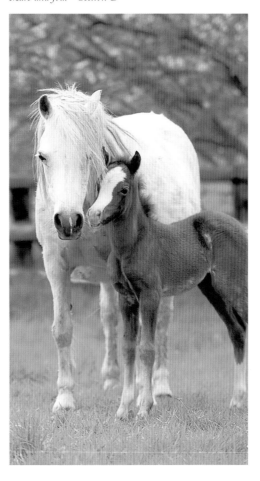

29

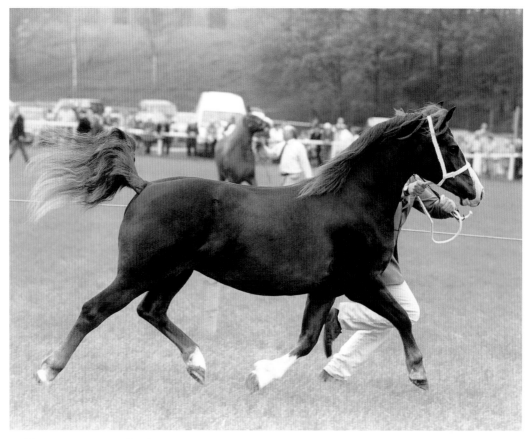

Welsh Section C mare Synod Lady Kate

The Welsh Pony of Cob Type – Section C

Height: Not exceeding 13.2hh.

The Welsh Pony of Cob type is the stronger counterpart of the Welsh Pony but with cob blood. The official description of this section is the same as that for Section D, the only difference being the lower height limit of the Section C.

The Welsh Cob – Section D

Height: There is no upper height limit, but until recently there was a height limit of 14.2hh for some ridden show classes. Cobs have therefore, in recent years, been bred to around this height.

General character: Strong, hardy and active with pony character and as much substance as possible.

Colour: Any colour, except piebald or skewbald.

Head: Must be full of quality and pony character – a coarse head and/or Roman nose are most objectionable. Ears should be bold and prominent and set widely apart; ears neat and well set.

Front: The neck should have a good length and be well carried. Moderately lean in the case of mares, but inclined to be cresty in the case of mature stallions. Shoulders should be strong but well laid back.

Forelegs: Set square and not tied in at the elbows. Long, strong forearms. Knees well developed with abundance of bone below the knee. Pasterns of proportionate slope and length. Feet well shaped and hooves dense. When in the rough, a moderate quantity of silky feather is acceptable, wiry hair is definitely unacceptable.

Middlepiece: Back and loins should be muscular and strong, and well coupled. Deep through heart and well ribbed up.

Hindquarters: Lengthy and strong. Ragged or drooping quarters are objectionable. Tail should be well set on.

Hind legs: Second thighs, strong and muscular. Hocks should be large, flat and clean with points prominent, turning neither inward nor outward. The hind legs must not be too bent, and the hock should be set behind a line falling from the point of the quarter to the fetlock joint. Pasterns of proportionate slope and length. Feet well shaped. Hooves dense.

Action: Free, true and forcible. The knee should be bent and the whole foreleg should be extended straight from the shoulder and as far forward as possible in the trot. Hocks must flex under the body with straight and powerful leverage.

Cathedine Express - Welsh Cob Section D

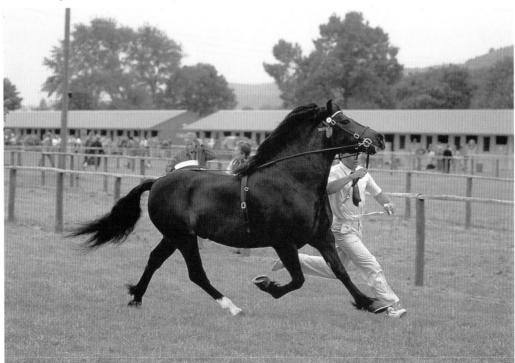

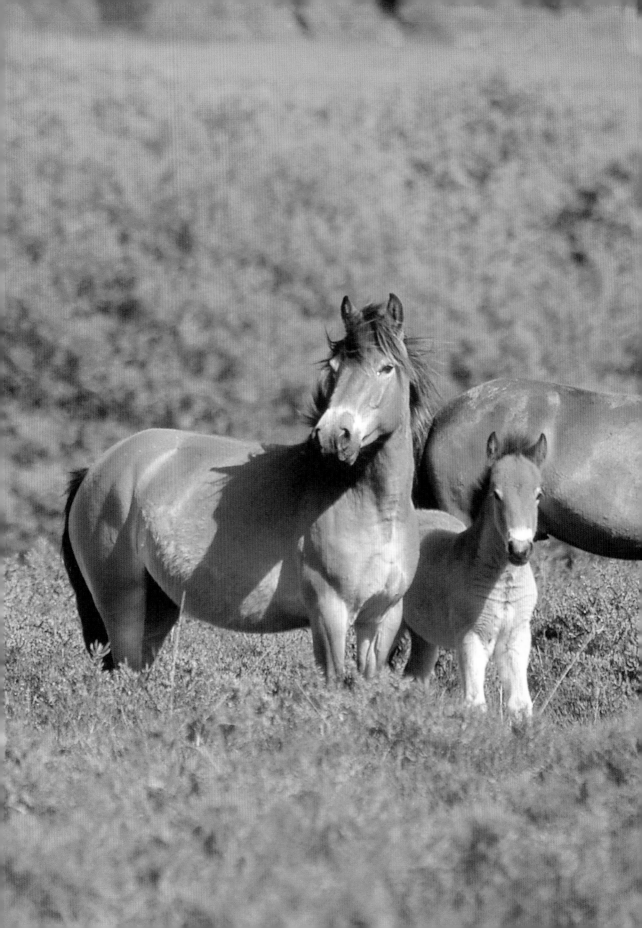

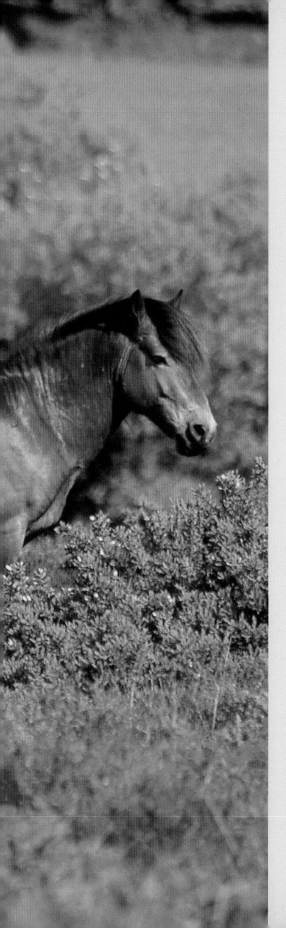

2

Accommodation

Never buy a horse or pony unless you have made suitable arrangements for his accommodation. You might think that it is easy to find grazing – after all there are fields everywhere – but for every farmer who does not mind horses there are ten who do not like them on their land. The usual possibilities for accommodation are as follows:

Livery Stables

There are various types of livery available.

FULL LIVERY

Here your horse either lives in fully or partly in and partly out and is cared for completely, including exercise and tack cleaning, by the stable staff. The advantage of this is that you only have to turn up when you want to ride and you can be sure (if you choose a good stable) that he will be cared for whatever you are doing. If you are ill or away from home on holiday or at work then he will always get appropriate care.

The main disadvantages of this system are that you do not form such a close relationship with your pony because you do not handle him all the time and the financial cost will be quite substantial.

PART LIVERY

This means that you will do some of the work but stable staff will do such jobs as are agreed for example turning out in the morning or feeding. This is cheaper but will mean a greater input from you. However, it usually means that your pony can be stabled at night especially in the winter.

GRASS LIVERY

This is the cheapest livery option. Your pony will live out in the field, although he may be given feed and/or hay by staff if this is agreed. Most natives are quite happy doing this and if he is kept at a stables there will be staff around to keep an eye on him when you are not there. There may also be the use of a stable if he is ill or lame.

Your own accommodation

If you have paddocks and/or stables at home, then you will be saved livery costs. However, you may find that it is difficult to go away on holiday unless you can arrange livery or have someone who can come in and look after your pony for you. You should have a minimum of one acre per horse. If your garden adjoins your paddocks then you should take special care to read the section in this chapter on poisonous plants. Many poisonings occur because

ponies lean over and eat garden plants. Garden plants can also seed themselves into adjoining land.

Rented grazing and/or stabling

This should be near enough to your home to ensure that travelling in bad weather is not a problem. You should ensure that you have a written agreement with the landowner, giving details of such matters as rent payable; amount of notice needed (on both sides) and responsibility for fencing, water supplies and possible damage. A pony kept away from home must be visited at least twice a day. It may be possible to enlist the help of neighbours to the field who could telephone you if they are worried.

Grazing

Native ponies have evolved through many generations to live in the very poorest conditions. It is only relatively recently in the scheme of things, say in the last hundred years or so, that we have been keeping the majority of our ponies on lusher lowland pasture. It is not surprising therefore that even in a small field a native pony can get very fat indeed when left to his own devices.

The very best grazing is old pasture land which has been well cared for by its previous owners. It should contain a variety of different grasses, together with such beneficial herbs as are listed on page 38. If a farmer has had cattle or sheep on a pasture he will have eradicated most of the

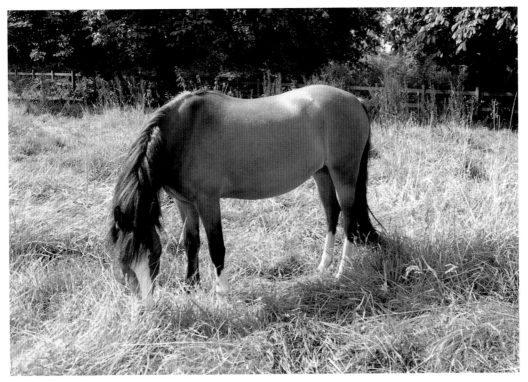

This field is unsuitable for pony grazing because of its proliferation of weeds, especially docks and rank long grasses

perennial weeds and will hopefully have also dealt with the poisonous ones too. Pasture which has been previously grazed by horses will benefit by resting for as long as possible. The best option here being to take a hay crop if the land can be left long enough and the time of year is right.

Grassland which has been previously arable land may have several problems. It may be too rich for ponies, having been fertilised for a previous crop. There may be plants of the previous crop growing through, such as oil seed rape, which is poisonous to horses. The land having been churned up by ploughing may well be more easily damaged than ground which has had many years to stabilise.

Land which has been left vacant for some reason can prove to be useful land for horses with some work. If the grass is long it would need to be 'topped'. This means cutting the grass and whatever else is growing there at a few inches long. The 'hay' can be left to dry, raked into heaps and burned. Do not save it to feed in case there are poisonous plants hidden in it. If you do not have a tractor and the necessary implements, some farmers will do the work – for a fee! Rubbish should be diligently removed and the ground checked for rabbit holes and other possible hazards. Poisonous plants can be removed by digging up and burning if there are not too many. Other weeds can be sprayed but care must be taken to observe all necessary precautions.

If you have a problem with ponies getting too fat there are several remedies. Firstly you can confine the pony in a small area. This can be done successfully with electric fencing. The fence can then be moved a few feet each day to give a limited area of new grazing. The field can be shared with sheep. It can be grazed by cattle or sheep first before the ponies. It can be regularly 'topped' and the excess gathered up and burnt.

Do remember however that on limited grazing many ponies become deficient in essential minerals. This is easily solved with a mineral lick or block.

COMMON POISONOUS PLANTS

Native ponies are usually careful to avoid poisonous plants. Their inbuilt 'dowsing' instinct is passed down from mare to foal and can protect them from danger. However, when we take our ponies away from their natural habitat and put them with plants which may not even be native species let alone 'wild' plants then occasionally mistakes can occur. Many poisonous plants have a bitter taste which will repel a well fed pony, but in bad weather or with insufficient grazing ponies may eat something which they would not normally consider. If you do not know what various plants look like then purchase a good guide book, with clear colour photographs (not drawings which are sometimes not accurate enough). Deal with offending plants by pulling up and burning if there are just a few, spraying if there is a vigorous growth and fencing off if it is a tree or hedge which cannot be moved or destroyed.

The list below contains the most usually found poisonous pasture.

COMMON POISONOUS PLANTS

- Beech (*Fagus sylvatica*). 300–500g (11–18oz) of the fruit (beech mast) are enough to poison fatally a horse.

- Box (*Buxus sempervirens*).

- Bracken (*Pteridium aquilinum*).

- Buttercup (*Ranunculus* species). Rarely eaten because the bitter taste is a deterrent. However, the taste is altered by weedkillers and it can then be eaten. Paddocks should be left at least fourteen days after treatment. Occasionally a skin allergy has been seen especially in pink-nosed horses grazing amongst buttercups.

- Daffodil (*Narcissus* species).

- Deadly Nightshade (*Atropa belladonna*). Can sometimes be eaten accidentally by animals browsing in the hedgerow. It is very dangerous. If you pull it out of your hedgerow, wear stout gloves. The sap can cause skin blistering.

- Foxglove (*Digitalis purpurea*). This is very common in paddocks and would not normally be eaten.

- Hemlock (*Conium maculatum*). This plant can be most dangerous in spring, when the young shoots are palatable to animals.

- Holly (*Ilex aquifolium*). The berries have proved poisonous particularly to young foals.

- Horse Chestnut (*Aesculus hippocastanum*). Horses can browse the leaves with no apparent ill effect. However consumption of the fruit (conkers) has occasionally proved fatal.

- Horseradish (*Amoracia rusticana*). The first part of the name is an old way of saying 'coarse' and does not mean a plant is good for or eaten by horses.

- Horsetail (*Equisetum* species).

- Ivy (*Hedera helix*). Dangerous if eaten in quantity.

- Laburnum (*Laburnum anagyroides*).

- Lupin (*Lupinus* species).

- Oak (*Quercus* species). The consumption of large quantities of acorns has proved fatal. Occasionally animals develop a craving for acorns. The reasons are not understood.

- Privet (*Ligustrum* species).

- Ragwort (*Senecio jacobaea*).

- Rhododendron (*Rhododendron ponticum*).

- Yew (*Taxus baccata*). Poisoning can be so sudden that the dead animal is found to still have the plant material in its mouth.

COMMON PERENNIAL WEEDS

These are weeds which although not particularly dangerous to grazing horses are nevertheless undesirable because they take up space and nutrients which would be better utilised by grass. Spraying with an appropriate herbicide is the only sure way to get rid of them.

COMMON PERENNIAL WEEDS

- Dock (*Rumex* species). There are various different members of the dock family but all are equally difficult to eradicate completely. Never let them go to seed – you will regret it ever after!

- Nettles (*Urtica* species). Nettles would actually be beneficial to horses if we could get them to eat them, but they never do! They have fairly shallow roots and small patches can be dug up and burnt.

• Plantain (*Plantago media*). Plantains spread along the ground putting up rosettes of leaves and tall thin 'flower' spikes looking similar to rushes. Each plant takes up space which could be better occupied by several grass plants.

• Rushes (*Juncus* species). Rushes are an indicator of sour wet pasture. After spraying with herbicide, attention should be given to drainage and liming of the land to improve the situation. Rushes can be notoriously difficult to get rid of. Cutting them down regularly can help the herbicide to work.

• Thistles (*Cirsium* species). Another persistent unwelcome guest and prolific seeder.

BENEFICIAL HERBS

These are plants which would naturally be present (or at least some of them) in old pasture. They would be eaten by ponies in the wild and are often relished by modern day ponies if they find a source. It is possible to buy wildflower seed mixes which have good herbs in them but they may also contain poisonous or unwanted ones. Do check the contents list. You can also gather seeds from your garden – especially easy for example in the case of dandelions – and broadcast sow them over your grass. This should be done as soon as the seeds are ripe as would happen in nature.

The following are well worth encouraging:

BENEFICIAL PLANTS

• Dandelion.

• Sow thistle.

• Beaked parsley also known as cow parsley, wild chervil and ketch.

• Hedge garlic.

• Chickweed.

• Lucerne.

• Furze also known as gorse.

• Red clover – but not too much for fat ponies!

• Bramble – but do not allow them free rein.

• Salad burnet.

• Dog rose.

• Goose grass also known as cleavers and sticky willie.

• Coltsfoot.

• Groundsel.

THE IDEAL FIELD

There is of course no such thing but certain characteristics are to be desired for keeping ponies. Old pasture which has been cut for hay in the past or grazed by cattle is always better than newly seeded land. There should be a good balance of plants. It does not need to be level or even flat for ponies but should be

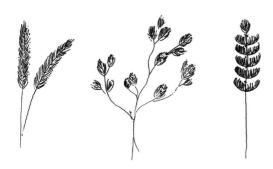

Common meadow grasses - timothy, red fescue, crested dogstail

safe. This means no steep slopes or sudden drops and no rocky outcrops which might prove hazardous. A good stout hedge especially to the windward side or a small spinney can provide good shelter. A field shelter with its back to the wind is even more desirable. Trees are useful for summer shade and provision should be available for watering. This should be either a trough or possibly a stream. Do however avoid sandy streams. Horses can ingest sand and become very ill from sand colic. If your stream is suspect, fence if off. It is always debatable as to whether it is safe to keep horses adjoining a motorway or very busy road. Not only are there the traffic fumes to consider but a traffic accident could leave you with a gap in the fence and your

ponies on the road. Ponies can also get excited and get through fencing.

It is also useful to consider whether or not your ponies would be seen if there is an emergency. If your field has no neighbours at all you will have to visit more often. If it has neighbours who would telephone you if there was a problem, it pays to make friends with them.

MAINTAINING YOUR GRAZING

If you only have a small area of grazing it makes very good sense to maintain it in good heart. If at all possible split it into at least two parts, so that one area can be resting whilst the other is being grazed. If you are lucky enough to have more grazing, you may well be able to make your own hay.

Make a point of walking all round the field at least once a week. Check the fencing and look out for anything which may cause harm to the pony such as litter thrown over the fence or dead branches falling. Check for holes, especially if you have rabbits in the area. A rabbit hole is much the same size as a pony's foot and a hole only a few inches deep can break an unlucky pony's leg.

Check for seedlings of poisonous plants. One of the very worst is ragwort and unfortunately its seeds blow about everywhere and seem to take hold very easily. Seedlings should be pulled up and burnt immediately. Other plants such as deadly nightshade and foxgloves can seed themselves from elsewhere and should receive the same treatment.

You will notice after a while in a new

field that the ponies are preferring some parts of the field and leaving others. These they will use as a toilet facility and this means that the grass there is useless.

If the field is small enough you can pick up the droppings with a shovel or fork and barrow. If it is larger you will need to have it harrowed regularly. A neighbouring farmer may do it for a fee or you can train your pony to pull a harrow and do it yourself. Failing all these options, you will have to scatter them yourself with a wire toothed rake.

Another task which needs to be done regularly is something called topping. This means cutting off any tall inedible grasses together with nettles and so on. Again you can call in a local farmer or contractor or you can hire a device called an Allenscythe which is a kind of heavy duty mower designed for rough ground. Check your ditches and keep them free from debris. This will have the added effect of making them easily visible to the ponies who are then less likely to injure themselves falling in.

If your field has areas which are constantly wet it is relatively simple to lay basic land drains yourself. Dig a trench about one foot (30cm) wide and running well away from the damp area in a downhill direction. Put about six inches (15cm) of coarse gravel and small pebbles in the bottom, refill and level.

Your field will need fertilizing after a while. This cannot really be done whilst being grazed. Take expert advice about what product to use but a useful tip is that seaweed based fertilisers seem to produce good grass for ponies which will not be too rich as is the risk with chemicals. Some stud owners also believe that the minerals in organic based fertilizers help to increase fertility.

The Agricultural Development and Advisory Service can help you ascertain exactly what is needed for your field at any time. Your local ADAS office will be listed in your telephone directory. If your ponies are eating bark or soil then there is almost certainly some deficiency in their diet.

It is important to re-seed bare areas if you are short of grazing. The easiest way to do this is to rake the surface lightly and scatter on a seed mixture which has been designed for horse paddocks. Rake it in and water if the weather is dry. There are certain grasses which are preferred by horses above others. Hybrid ryegrass; tall fescue; creeping red fescue and crested dogtail probably come in most ponies' first list. Highland bent grass is another variety often found in pony paddock mixtures.

Fencing

Fencing has to be adequate both to keep your horses in safely and to keep potential thieves out.

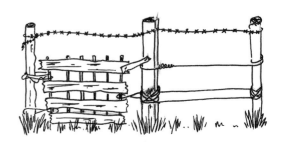

Unsuitable fencing for a pony

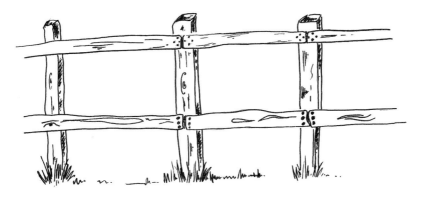

Post and rails

POST AND RAILS

This is always used when livestock is valuable and is always the fencing of choice. It is however, of course, the most expensive. A point to remember with native ponies is to ensure that the rails are close enough together and that the bottom of the rail is near enough to the ground. A determined Shetland or even one of the other small breeds can get under a rail if it is more than about two feet (61cm) off the ground. A Dartmoor pony, who shall remain nameless, could get easily between two rails just two feet three inches (70cm) apart. I am sure you get the picture now! Post and rails should be inspected regularly for broken rails or loose posts.

HEDGING

A good thick natural hedge makes a stout barrier and provides a natural windbreak. If possible, let the hedge on the side of the prevailing wind grow tall for this purpose. Hedges should be checked for poisonous plants and thin patches should be reinforced with a rail or two until they grow thicker. Trim back in the autumn, especially on the inside edges of the field. If you are short of grazing, much ground can be gained by keeping the hedges trimmed back where they belong. If you want to plant a new hedge or thicken up an existing one, the native species blackthorn and hawthorn work well, as well as being harmless if they are eaten. Strands of blackberry can be woven in to your hedge by a brave person wearing stout gloves. As well as strengthening the hedge, the young shoots are universally adored by ponies. If you have ornamental species such as privet or laurel or yew in your hedge or anything you cannot identify, you are best to dig it up and burn it rather than risk poisoning. Native ponies will sometimes eat herbage that they would normally ignore if they are on restricted grazing or have run out of hay in the winter.

WIRE

Barbed wire is an absolute disaster with ponies. It is just not safe and should be avoided at all costs. Sometimes, three strands of wire stretched between posts can work as a cheap fencing, but it must be kept very taut and should be good heavy duty wire, as thick as you can get. Make sure that the bottom strand is not low enough to get a leg over – or indeed high enough so as not to tempt an escape. It is possible now to buy fencing 'tape', which is similar to electric fencing tape and can be stretched taut between posts. It is much more visible than wire.

ELECTRIC FENCING

This is a good temporary solution to a number of problems but should never be considered permanent. Electric fencing is very useful for restricting grazing and for overweight animals a strip grazing system can be employed. This is where access to a limited amount of extra grazing is allowed each day without having to let the pony into a whole new field. Ensure that the fence is set up correctly, according to the manufacturer's instructions and that the posts are firmly set into the ground. Electric fencing can also be useful to mend gaps in the hedge temporarily; to keep ponies away from muddy areas in winter and to keep two new animals apart whilst they get to know each other.

Electric fencing is useful for dividing a large field

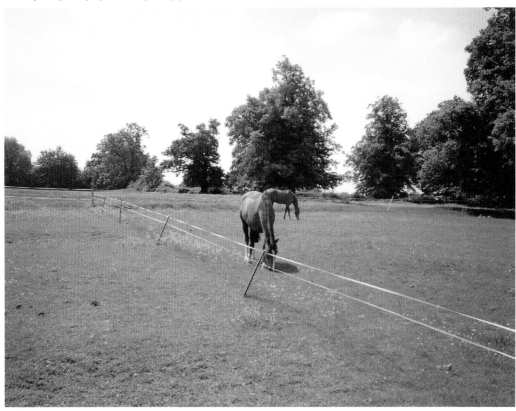

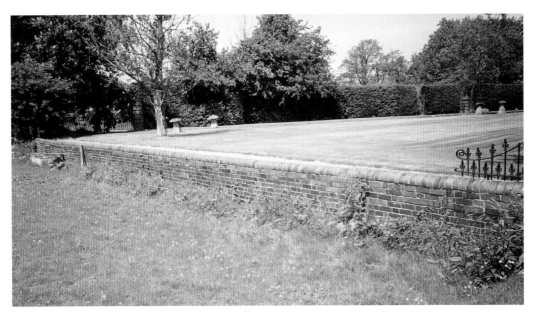

This is a ha-ha, but beware of native ponies spotting the grass on the top!

OTHER FENCING

It is possible to use all sorts of things as fencing for horses – I have seen everything from old bedsteads to wooden pallets being used, with varying success. At the end of the day, you are well advised to buy the best you can afford and to maintain it well, rather than spend all your spare time patching up a mish-mash of fencing which will never really be totally successful.

Gates

You will need a gate which is wide enough to take a tractor for maintenance work and it can also be useful to have a small gate, just large enough to take ponies in and out to save opening the main gate. Ponies often stand near to the gate and the area can become muddy very quickly in winter. This can be solved by putting down hardcore in this area or by constructing a fence and a second gateway a few yards inside the field. This option can provide a useful area to separate one pony from others, for example if it is to be ridden and can also guard against a mass exodus when you only want to remove one animal from the field. It will of course add to your costs, but is well worth thinking about from a practical point of view. Always feed animals well away from the gate to avoid adding to poaching of the ground there.

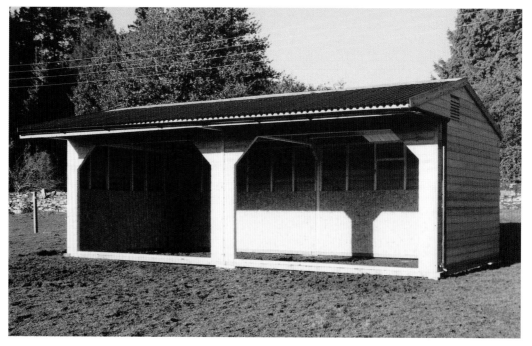

Field shelter

Field Shelters

An open fronted oblong timber shed is the most usual type of field shelter. The only considerations are that it is of safe construction and that it has no corners or other areas where a pony might get trapped if there is a disagreement. You can usefully bed down a shelter with straw or shavings and provide a cosy place where ponies who are out all winter can lie down. However, do not be disappointed if you build a beautiful shelter and the pony ignores it. Some ponies do not bother to shelter.

Watering Arrangements

A good clean source of water supply is essential. The very best solution is a trough fed directly from the water mains and filled by means of a ball-cock system which ensures that the amount of water in the trough is kept up to an agreed level. This is not always possible especially if the field is rented and in that case a trough of some sort must be installed, and filled manually. Rubber troughs are good, being less likely to cause injury. However, they are less long lasting than galvanised metal or cast iron. It is possible to use an old bath, but the taps should be removed to avoid injury. The plug hole can be useful for draining and cleaning but any plug chain should be removed.

Water troughs can easily go green and smelly in hot weather and should be checked every day in cold weather in case ice has formed. Self-filling troughs will need careful protection from frost. Whatever your arrangements the basic rule of thumb is that every pony should have access to clean fresh water at all times, day and night.

Security

Horsewatch schemes are a brilliant idea. Join your local group if you have one. They will give you valuable advice about security and can provide warning notices and other devices to help avoid a potential theft.

If your field gate is near enough to your house for an alarm to be heard if the gate is opened by an unauthorised person it is worth buying a gate alarm. Failing this, buy a stout lock and chain and train yourself to keep it locked at all times. If the gate is the kind with lift off hinges, you should also padlock and chain the hinge end to prevent the gate being opened by lifting it off the hinges.

Freezemarking is a tricky subject where native ponies are concerned and particularly if you want to show your pony. Judges are told not to take notice of freezemarking but they do still seem to do so and this seems to happen more in in-hand classes rather than in ridden ones. However, if you live in a high risk area or are at all worried then you should either freezemark and take no notice of whatever anyone else says, or go for branding of hooves with your postcode or investigate such solutions as lip tattooing.

If your pony is wearing a rug, you can write on it with a permanent marker pen, in big letters 'PONY FREEZEMARKED UNDER RUG', whether it is or not. Only the most determined thief would bother to take the rug off to check.

Unless your pony is desperately difficult to catch you should not leave a headcollar on. It not only makes theft more easy but it could get caught up in the hedge or fence with potentially serious consequences. If you have a pen inside the gate (see 'gates' on page 43) you will always be able to herd a difficult to catch pony into the gateway pen and make him easier to get hold of without risking leaving his headcollar on.

Your tack is very valuable too. Never leave it in the yard or even somewhere in the field. It should always be locked up, preferably in your house. It should also be postcoded or otherwise marked so that you can identify it. Rugs too should not be left lying around for opportunist thieves.

Stables

Stables come in all shapes and sizes and are built out of every conceivable material. However, if you are building stables from scratch then there are some points to consider. The most important is that you will almost certainly need planning permission. Your local council will give you all the details.

You will need to think about the size of your stables. The larger breeds will obviously need more room. You might

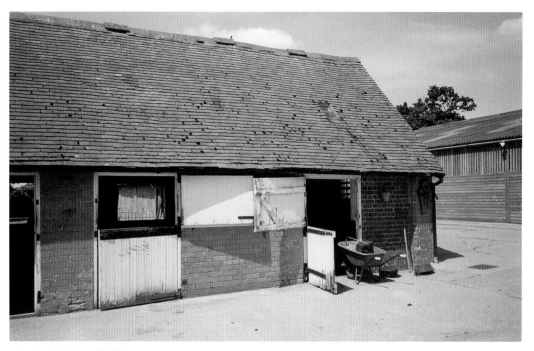

A lovely old brick stable block

have a Shetland now but will your children be growing and moving onto larger animals? You can put a small pony in a big stable but not the other way round. Which way does the wind most frequently come from? If your stables are rained in on every time there is bad weather you will waste bedding. You will need a concrete or other firm material area outside the stables. Do not forget to allow for this in your plans.

Around eight feet (2.5m) square or thereabouts is sufficient for the small breeds but this should be at least ten feet (3m) square for a Welsh Section C or New Forest and twelve feet (3.9m) square for a Welsh Cob or Highland. The roof height and height of the door lintel should be sufficient to prevent injury. The whole area of a stable should allow for enough air to circulate. An outside stable needs 1600 cubic feet (45 cubic metres) of air for your horse to be kept in good health. The more air available the better. Ponies often start to have wind problems when they are confined in stuffy stables and fed dusty hay or otherwise bad hay.

The most common materials for building new stables are as follows:

Brick: This is expensive but long lasting.
Concrete Block: Cheaper than brick but not quite so pleasing to look at. Can be improved by rendering.
Wood: Timber stables can be bought easily in pre-fabricated form. They will not last as long as brick but can be aesthetically pleasing, especially if well maintained. Timber does have a slightly increased fire risk.

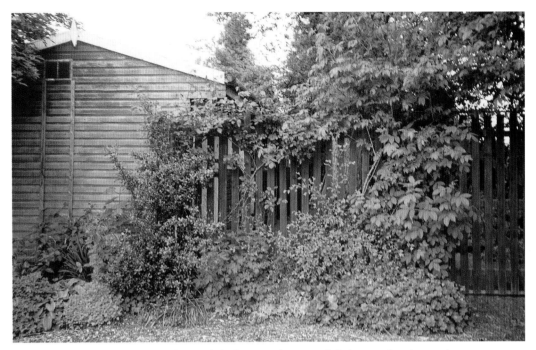

This stable block is protected by a high fence with climbing roses (roses are safe for horses and ponies to eat)

Barn or indoor stables are wonderful for a big yard, especially in bad weather. If the partitions are too low, you run a risk of bullying and there is always an increased risk of infection passing on more easily.

Stables can be built on compacted earth. For small ponies this can work very well, especially if your soil is free draining. However, most stable floors are concrete for ease of cleaning. Provision must be made for drainage, in accordance with local planning regulations. Thought must also be given to storm water drainage, by way of roof guttering.

The walls of your stable can be covered at least half way up with suitable material for kicking boards. These give a pony something to push against when he is getting up and avoid injuries such as capped hocks. For valuable ponies rubber lining for stables gives the best protection. Lining the walls also helps to strengthen and insulate wooden walls.

Roofing can be in any number of materials and can incorporate clear perspex sheeting for extra light. Galvanised metal is not recommended because it gets very hot in good weather and thatch is not recommended because of the increased fire risk.

Windows should not be of glass unless adequately protected on the inside with stick-on clear plastic. Perpex is acceptable but both should be protected with a metal grid. A metal grid alone can be used. Bars are not safe because of the risk of a pony putting his head or foot through them and getting trapped.

Doorways should be at least eight feet (2.4m) high and four feet (1.2m) wide. A door seven feet (2m) high and three feet six inches (1.1m) wide is enough for ponies. The

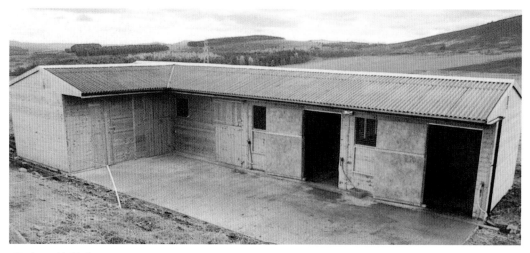

Wooden stable block

bottom door should ideally be in proportion to the size of the pony. If your pony has to crane his neck all the time to see over the door he will develop unwanted muscles on the underside of his neck. There should be no gap between the bottom of the door and the floor. A gap allows draughts and a gap bigger than a few inches would allow a foot to get trapped. The door edge should be protected from chewing with a metal strip. Do not use lead roofing strip which is poisonous. Top doors are useful for bad weather but not essential. There should be some method (usually a hook and eye) for securing the door open when mucking out and so on. There will need to be two bolts on the door at top and bottom or a bolt at the top and kick-over latch at the bottom. Never ever padlock shut the bolts on a stable door. It might seem like a good safety precaution but in the event of a fire or other emergency it can stop quick rescue.

There should be a ring to tie a horse up inside and to tie a haynet to if you use one. Built-in mangers can save effort at feeding time but can also cause injury. One solution can be a temporary manger put over the stable door and removed after feeding. They can be too high for small ponies to feed comfortably. Bucket rings are to be avoided at all costs. They are the very easiest way for a horse to injure his legs.

Watering can be done from a solid heavy bucket in the corner of the stable or from a built-in automatic system. There are pros and cons for both: buckets mean filling, emptying and washing out and automatic systems can freeze in winter and will not be used by shy ponies.

Lighting is best done by electricity and installed by a competent electrician. Switches should be proper ones for outdoor use and installed high up on the outside of the stables. The wires should run in metal piping installed out of horses' reach. The light itself, whether fluorescent tube or light bulb should be placed well out of reach up in the roof. Outside lights should be bulkhead lights for outside use installed at strategic points around the yard. It is possible to get security lights which come on when movement is detected to deter thieves. A power point is also useful in the yard to operate clippers and so on. Horses are more easily electrocuted than humans and therefore every care should be taken to avoid any risk.

A stable designated for washing is very useful. It should have a good drain in the centre and a water supply laid on. Heat lamps for drying ponies after exercise and bathing are a real bonus. If this is not possible, then an area can be set aside outside for bathing with a good drain and a tap nearby.

Your stable yard will also need a vermin-proof facility for storing feed and somewhere to store your hay and bedding. Storing hay in an area which shares the same roof space as the stables used for horses can cause hay allergies.

The surface of the yard can be of various materials with concrete or tarmac being the most expensive but the easiest to keep clean. You may want to consider other matters such as the parking of a lorry or trailer when designing your layout.

Bedding for stables

STRAW

Straw is the most common medium for horse bedding. It is usually cheap and easy to obtain. Wheat straw is preferable as ponies tend to eat both oat and barley straw. Straw produces a larger muckheap than anything else, but it can sometimes be sold to mushroom growers and others. It is also bulky to store. Good straw is shiny and clean with no dust or mould.

WOOD SHAVINGS

Shavings are ideal for ponies with a dust allergy. They can also be the bedding of choice if you only have room for a small muckheap. If you are very lucky you might be able to obtain them free of charge from a local timber yard, but do take care to avoid hardwood shavings and any which might have nails or other debris. Purchased shavings come in plastic covered bales which can be stored outside if necessary.

PAPER

Shredded paper is warm and comfortable but can be expensive. It rots down easily so providing a small heap but before it starts to rot it does blow about in the yard easily. This can be solved to some extent by hosing the muck heap. Paper bales too can be stored outside.

HEMP

This is a relative newcomer to the horse bedding field. It looks like finely chopped straw and is very easy and tidy to use. It is however expensive and can sometimes be difficult to obtain.

RUBBER MATTING

Rubber mats are sold as being easy to use without any bedding at all. It seems somewhat callous to expect ponies with all their protruding bony bits to lie down on a rubber mat with no bedding. Where these mats do come into their own is when used with an area of bedding to lie down on. The pony can then stand on rubber and not concrete when feeding and so on. This can be very beneficial for old ponies and others with leg problems.

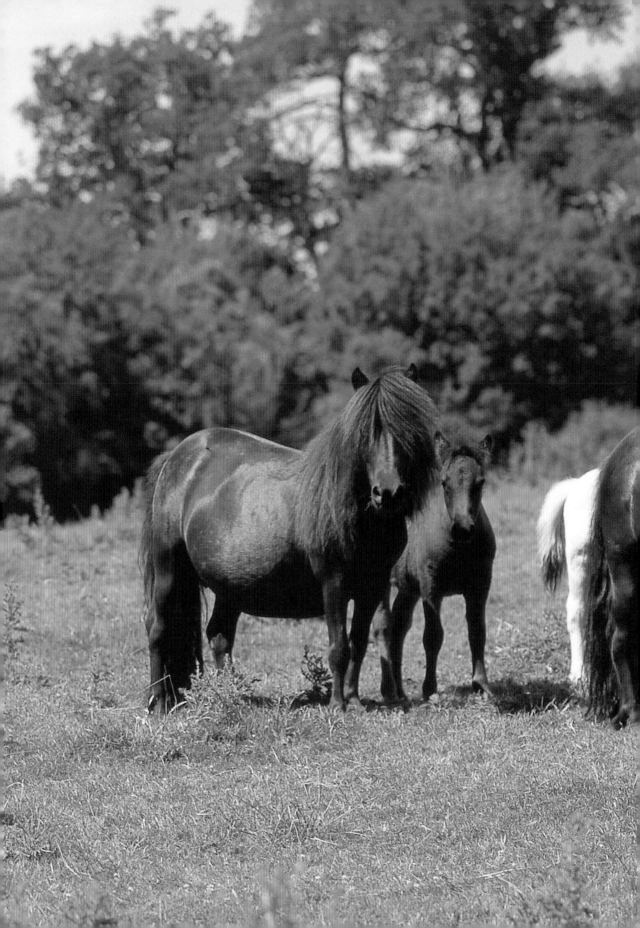

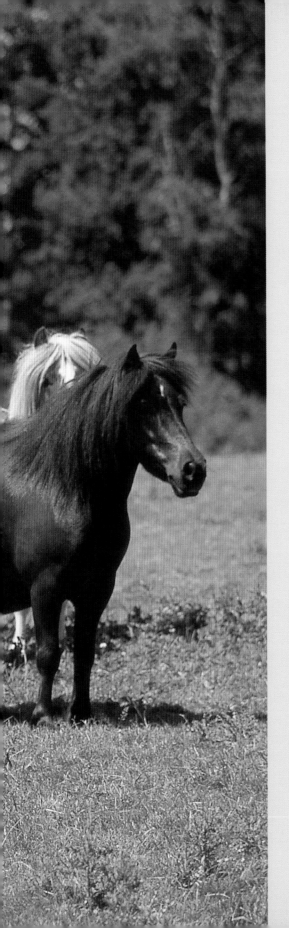

3

Feeding

It is a common fallacy that native ponies can live almost on fresh air. Ponies are seen on Dartmoor and in places on the Welsh hills where there is little or no grass and they appear to be eating just gorse and other odd bits of greenery and doing very well. It is conveniently forgotten that many of them die in a hard winter despite the fact that farmers and owners put out supplementary food. They would also not be in optimum condition for competition or showing, using all their energy in searching for more food and other survival necessities. So how did ponies originally survive in the wild, you might ask? The answer is that they roamed much further afield. There was much less 'farming' of land and certainly far less road traffic and other modern hazards. There was therefore food available over a much wider area and therefore in effect, more food. We also, of course did not ride these ponies, let alone get them to undertake such arduous tasks as jumping, hunting and other equestrian sports.

The other important point to consider today is that we have substantially

A group of Shetland Ponies at Stepney Stud   51

weakened the in-built hardiness of our native ponies by keeping successive generations in a much 'softer' lifestyle. We have changed both their diet and their expectations. Conversely, by doing this we have also in effect introduced disorders such as laminitis, which the residue of their wild heritage makes them more prone to!

A and fit healthy native pony can still live outdoors all the year round, providing he has adequate shelter and supplementary feeding in bad weather. For ponies already grown and doing no work this can just be good hay. A horse or pony is designed for most of his diet to be bulk fibre and for most of his digestive system to be occupied at any one time. For this reason the old maxim of feeding little and often is a good one. At grass, the average pony eats almost constantly, so that when a horse is stabled he needs to have almost constant access to bulk forage (and of course to water). For this reason hay is a most important subject in any modern pony's life.

Hay

There are basically three types of hay. These are seed hay, meadow hay and haylage.

Seed hay is grown on land which has been ploughed up and re-seeded especially to grow a hay crop. The actual grasses in it depend on the type(s) sown, but usually this includes rye which produces a hard 'stalky' grass, together with other less sturdy grasses and possibly clover. The resulting hay is hard in texture; often seeming to be all stalks and is best when slightly green coloured. Horses almost

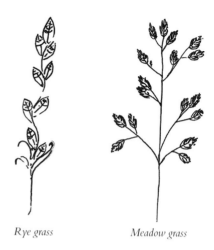

Rye grass   *Meadow grass*

universally love seed hay, however it is usually too high in protein for native ponies, except for breeding stock. However, it should also be said that poorly made seed hay can have less nutritional value than well-made meadow hay.

Meadow hay is grown on fields which already have grass established. These fields may have been used for grazing the previous year or may be used for a hay crop every summer and then used for grazing throughout the winter. Meadow hay is infinitely variable. It is nearly always softer in texture than seed hay and will contain various herbs and weeds. It can also contain dangerous plants such as ragwort and unpalatable plants such as thistles and docks. Hay from a new source should always be checked very carefully for undesirable plants and rejected completely if any evidence is found.

The quality of all hay depends on the actual grasses and other plants that it contains; the stage of growth at which it was cut; the weather and other factors during the drying process and the way in which it has been stored since harvesting.

It is possible, but expensive, to get the protein content of your hay checked but a practised eye works almost as well. Break open a bale and smell the hay. It should remind you of summer meadows, smelling sweet and fresh. If the smell is musty or damp or smelling of mushrooms, this is not good hay. There might be some loss of seeds as the bale opens but there should not be visible clouds of dust or anything else to make you sneeze. Then examine the hay carefully for anything undesirable, this includes things such as cow pats and bits of string or other debris, as well as the plants mentioned above. Lastly, look at the outside of the bale for areas of black hay. This is the result of the bale being stored somewhere and rain getting in. This part of the bale can be discarded if the rest is good, but a bale with a black side, for example, should be discarded altogether.

There is also a process which occurs when hay is too damp when it is baled. The haystack heats up and in effect finishes the drying off of the contents. The hay will be brown in colour and have a smell, which is something like beer. Whilst this hay is still safe to feed, it will be of a poorer quality.

Hay should be stored in dry conditions with adequate ventilation. Stacking bales on pallets allows for a good airflow around the bales.

It is said that new hay should not be fed until the New Year. However, this is not always possible particularly in recent poor summers, when hay is in short supply by the time the next crop is cut. If feeding new hay, do not use it if it is hot to touch, because fermentation is taking place and the result would be indigestion.

Dusty hay can cause enormous problems both to your pony and to you. Chronic Obstructive Pulmonary Disease (COPD) occurs when poor quality, mouldy hay is fed and the pony develops a sensitivity to the mould spores and also to the forage mites which live in mouldy hay (and concentrates). Hay can be soaked or steamed to lessen the risk. There is some controversy about the length of time that hay should be soaked for. It used to be thought that it was imperative to soak the hay overnight. Now it is generally thought that this just makes the hay slimy and unpalatable. Recent research shows that six minutes is long enough for the hay to be immersed in *clean* water in a clean dustbin or other vessel. The water will need to be dripped out by hanging the haynet in a suitable place, before feeding to the pony. In freezing conditions you can soak the hay in hot water and this will help to stop the hay freezing before the poor pony gets round to eating it all.

Steaming is accomplished by putting the haynet in a suitable utensil – it is possible to use a stout, clean polythene bag. Two or three kettles of boiling water are poured over and the bag or bin is sealed. The hay is left for an hour or so. Check carefully that it is cold before feeding – the inside of the hay will always be hotter than the outside and therefore this is where you should check.

Farmer's lung is a human condition which is not unlike broken wind or Chronic Obstructive Pulmonary Disease and is similarly caused by the spores in hay. Asthmatics and people with other lung problems should always wear a mask when dealing with hay.

Haylage

Haylage is grass which is cut slightly sooner than ordinary hay (but not cut as soon in the growth cycle as silage). It is not left to dry out completely as hay should be but is baled whilst not quite dry into bales which are then sealed with polythene, so that they are airtight. The grass ferments slightly in the bale, so that it ends up being something between hay and silage. This almost always ends up being a product which is higher in protein than hay and great care should therefore be taken in feeding it to native ponies, especially those prone to laminitis.

Haylage does, however, have some advantages over hay. It does not ever need to be soaked and can be fed without preparation to a pony with COPD. It is nearly always relished by horses and ponies and can tempt a fussy feeder or a pony who is or has been ill. If you have limited space, the bales are smaller than hay bales and can be stored outside.

Haylage can go mouldy inside the bale, especially if there is damage, even a tiny pinprick, in the outside wrapper. If this happens it should be discarded. However, an almost alcoholic smell and/or a white bloom are just related to the yeasts activated by the production method and are nothing to worry about.

A rough guide to the amount of haylage that should be fed is to feed an equal weight to the amount of hay that would otherwise be used. This is however a rough guide and dependent on such factors as the quality of hay previously fed and what else makes up the pony's diet. As with any new feed the changeover to haylage should be done gradually and the pony monitored carefully for signs of laminitis or colic.

Straw

For fat native ponies, a portion of their bulk ration can be good quality barley or wheat straw. It is harder to chew and can slow down the digestion of the rest of the hay ration. It also has few nutrients but plenty of fibre; this again can be useful for fat ponies. The only downside of using straw as a food is that it can encourage bed eating. Most ponies will eat some of their bed – some will eat so much that they have bare floor in the morning. If you have a bed eater you may just have to change to a less appetising bedding such as wood shavings.

FEEDING HAY

For ponies eating their hay ration in a stable, the hay can be put in a manger or haynet or fed on the floor. There are advantages and disadvantages to each method. Ponies can injure themselves on a fixed manger as with any other fittings in the stable. It is possible for a lively pony to get his foot caught in a haynet if it is not tied up high enough. Both of these methods encourage an unnatural feeding position. Feeding on the floor is the natural way, but a wasteful pony can spread hay everywhere and trample it into the bed before he pees on it making a dreadful mess. For a pony who has to stand in the stable for a long time it is possible to buy haynets with very small holes thus making the process of getting at the hay take longer and help to alleviate boredom.

Feeding hay in the field is always wasteful. It gets trampled into the mud and therefore becomes inedible. However, if you have ponies out all the time and bad weather sets in you will have to be prepared to waste some hay! It is not wise to use haynets because a pony caught up in the net could be there all night in cold weather with dire consequences. Hayracks designed for cattle are a possibility but if the rack is high the hayseeds can get into pony's eyes and the feeding position will be unnatural. A lower rack means that a pony could get a leg into it.

Feeding concentrates

READY PREPARED MIXES

These are the chosen feeds for many people nowadays. They are scientifically designed for various categories of equines, so that they receive an optimum diet. There are feeds on the market for old ponies, bloodstock, competition ponies, ponies who have had laminitis and so on and so on. They are quick and easy to feed and include vitamins and minerals so need possibly only the addition of some chaff to stop bolting.

The downside of mixes is that they are usually well coated in molasses that may provide too much sugar and may also encourage the pony to bolt the feed.

CUBES

Cubes too come in lots of different formulas. They are easy to feed but by the very nature of the presentation are dry and therefore possibly unpalatable to a fussy eater. Care should be taken that ponies do not bolt cubes which, being dry, cause a choke. Do this by feeding mixed into chaff.

Since both mixes and cubes provide a complete diet it is not advisable to add other grains (apart from a small amount of chaff) or food items and supplements should definitely not be added.

Other foods

OATS

Oats have a bad reputation that they do not deserve. Everyone knows such expressions as 'too much oats' to describe a lively pony. However oats are high in fibre and have hardly any more protein than barley and therefore it can be a very good food for ponies. They are especially good for the slow, possibly older pony whose little rider needs a bit of help before their legs drop off from too much kicking. It may be that some individuals have sensitivity to oats and become unmanageable on them. If you want to try oats, then introduce them slowly until you gauge your pony's reaction. Bloodstock for whom rideability is not an issue can do very well indeed on oats.

Naked oats are not suitable for ponies, except perhaps for the larger stallion. They are very high in protein.

Because the husk is hard to chew, oats

are better fed crushed but it should be borne in mind that they 'go off' quickly once they are crushed. Boiled oats can tempt a sick pony to eat.

BARLEY

Barley is often used for fattening ponies. It is very palatable when fed boiled; boiling also increases the digestibility. The hull of barley seeds is tightly attached to the grain and therefore barley must be crimped or rolled for it to be digestible. Barley has a high energy value and can be easy to overfeed and also to produce an allergic type reaction which shows as lumpy swellings or as filling in the legs.

MAIZE

Maize is usually only seen in ready mixes. It is expensive and can be heating and is therefore only worth buying as a single grain to feed to very poor doers.

LINSEED

Linseed is a brilliant conditioner and appetiser. It is usually bought as the 'raw' grain which must be cooked for several hours in plenty of water before feeding.

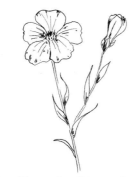

Linseed is a good conditioner and appetiser

When it is properly cooked it will jellify as it cools and can then be fed to ponies at the rate of a cupful or two of jelly per day. Overfeeding can cause diarrhoea. This action can be put to good use if your pony is constipated for any reason – although constipation is very rare in any grass fed animal and should therefore be a reason for concern. Linseed can sometimes be purchased as ready-made cake, but beware of feeding linseed cake designed for cattle. It is not suitable for horses.

SOYA

Soya can be very good food for horses but is very high in protein. For this reason it is best reserved for breeding stock especially mares when feeding a foal.

SUGAR BEET

Sugar beet is a very underrated food. It is cheap, easy to feed and generally relished. However, it is vital that sugar beet is soaked for twenty-four hours before feeding. It should never be fed dry. The bucket or whatever is used for soaking should be cleaned every day and refilled with clean water. In hot weather soaked sugar beet goes off very quickly and should be thrown away, especially if it is attracting flies. Sugar beet encourages fussy feeders and gives energy (because of its high sugar content) to sick or recovering ponies. It is also high in fibre and very useful for sustaining endurance horses and ponies competing all day at a show or event who may have to go without food for several hours.

Fillers

CHAFF

Chaff is chopped hay and/or straw and nowadays often contains alfalfa. Alfalfa increases the quality of chaff which would otherwise often be made from poor quality hay, well coated in molasses to make it palatable. Indeed most chaff is actually high in sugar because of the addition of molasses. However, you can now get low sugar products often called 'light' and these are more suitable for native ponies. Chaff can help to bulk out a feed for a greedy eater without giving him too much protein and adds fibre to the diet of ponies on restricted grazing.

BRAN

Bran used to be a very good addition to feed for ponies but modern milling methods have reduced the bran left to something with very little food value at all. It can therefore be useful, again, for overweight animals and greedy feeders. A bran mash can be very comforting for a sick or very tired animal. Put a couple of scoops of bran into a clean bucket with a good tablespoonful of salt. Add boiling water to make a fairly stiff porridge consistency. Allow to cool to blood heat before feeding. The addition of a little soaked sugar beet can be useful and appetising.

Supplements

If you are feeding a complete mix, then supplements should *not* be fed. If you are mixing your own food then you may need to add a complete vitamin and mineral mix (also known as a balancer) of which there are various ones on the market, again designed for different categories of pony. If you are mixing your own food and you have bloodstock or elderly ponies or animals with arthritis or laminitis then you may need a specialised supplement. If you live in a part of the country where there is a selenium or other mineral deficiency then you will need to add the appropriate mineral supplement. If you have any doubts then consult your local Agricultural Development and Advisory Service advisor or your vet. Do not feed minerals unless you are sure your pony needs them because an excess of any particular mineral can either be toxic or will just be excreted thus wasting money.

If you are feeding mostly grains then you will need a balanced calcium and phosphorus supplement. Bonemeal is the ideal way to feed this, but care should be taken to obtain sterilised bonemeal, properly packaged for feeding to horses.

Other additions to feed

OIL

Quite a high proportion of a pony's energy requirements can be met by oil. The type of oil given is usually just supermarket vegetable oil or sunflower seed oil, although there are some specialist ones coming on to the market lately. A teacupful a day is about the maximum you should feed and as with everything else it should be introduced gradually. Avoid oils that have been chemically processed, using pure ones and not those which have any other ingredients (such as chemicals to make them so that they do not stick to food).

SALT

The average pony's diet does not include enough salt. Signs of salt deficiency are licking or eating bark and soil, although ponies can be deficient without showing these signs. The best answer is to provide a salt lick or to add one tablespoonful of table salt to his daily feed.

CARROTS AND OTHER VEGETABLES

Ponies universally love carrots and apples. Carrots should be cut into long fingers, never into round slices. Apples can just be quartered. Ponies can also be fed swede and parsnip, again cut into long fingers and pears cut into quarters. Peelings from all of these can also be fed. Horses used to be fed potato peelings as a cure for broken wind but I have yet to find a pony who will eat them.

BREAD

Bread should never be fed to ponies without baking it to a dry crisp first. Unbaked bread can choke a pony.

Herbs and their uses

Herbs can provide a very useful addition to your pony's diet. After all, in the wild a much greater variety of herbage would have been eaten as ponies travelled relatively extensively on their search for food. It is also recognised that wild ponies have a 'dowsing' instinct, which means that they instinctively sought out certain plants when experiencing specific problems. This has largely been eradicated by domestication, but native ponies still retain more of this instinct than Thoroughbreds and others. Herbs are always best fed fresh if available, but should not be gathered from a possibly polluted source such as the roadside. It is always important to be absolutely sure of the identification of any plant that you want to feed to your pony. If you are not sure then buy it dried from a reputable supplier.

The following are some herbs which the amateur can safely use and which can be relatively easily identified:

GARLIC

Possibly the best known herb for feeding to horses. It is easily available in powdered form or can be fed as fresh cloves if your pony will eat them. Garlic has many uses, the most important being as an antibiotic,

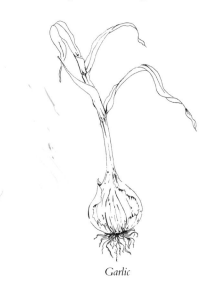

Garlic

expectorant and anti-parasitic. This means that it is helpful in any condition where there is bacterial infection (although it is not a substitute for antibiotics in serious infection); it is a useful adjunct to veterinary treatment in cases of respiratory infection and garlic can also help to keep down the level of worm infestation (although regular worming is still necessary). Since garlic also has a blood cleansing action it can be very useful in laminitis, sweet itch and other common native pony problems. In short it may well be the best advice to feed a measure of garlic to every equine, every day!

NETTLE

Everyone knows the stinging nettle. It grows anywhere where soil is disturbed and therefore is always around in stable yards, especially around the muckheap. Interestingly, ponies are very rarely seen to eat nettles, yet they can benefit from being fed them for a number of conditions. A blood cleansing effect means that laminitis,

sweet itch and other conditions which require 'cooling' can be helped by nettle. The iron content makes nettles a useful addition to veterinary treatment in cases of anaemia. Broodmares do well on nettles, the herb helping to boost milk production whilst giving a useful vitamin and mineral boost. As already mentioned, nettles do not seem to be palatable fresh, so you will need to gather them for your pony and dry them before adding to the feed. A handful of the dried matter would be the maximum dose.

DANDELION

Although seen as a nuisance when appearing in the lawn, dandelions should be positively encouraged in pony pasture. They are much loved by ponies who eat them down to the root and therefore will not allow them to spread too far. Dandelions are a very good liver tonic and

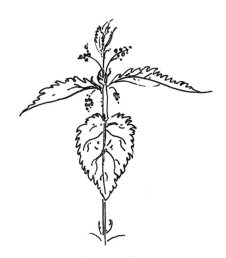

Stinging nettle

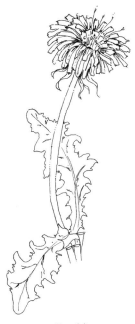

Dandelion

should be fed to every sick horse to help him with his recovery. They are especially useful if, as part of his veterinary treatment, he requires painkillers. Some painkillers are not the best news that your pony's liver ever had and therefore feeding dandelions at the rate of a handful dried or as many fresh leaves as he will eat will help to lessen the side-effects of the painkiller.

MINT
Ponies love mints. However, mints designed for human consumption contain a high proportion of sugar and in crunching the sweet the sugar is deposited on the pony's teeth. Horses get dental cavities in just the same way that humans do, but of course much more rarely since the bulk of their diet is *not* refined sugar. It is best therefore to keep mint sweets for a very occasional treat. Mint, though can be fed in other ways to good effect. Fussy feeders and those prone to digestive disturbance can be helped by a teaspoonful of dried or a dessertspoonful of fresh mint every day. A colicky pony who is to receive a bran mash can have the mash made with peppermint tea – put two peppermint tea bags in a pint of water. Fresh mint leaves can be rubbed on the itching of sweet itch or insect bites but not once the skin is broken.

MARIGOLD
Marigolds do not generally grow wild in Britain but can easily be grown in pots or elsewhere and can be a very attractive plant to grow in the stable yard where they might get eaten, since they pose no threat. The petals are used for liver problems internally and for fungal or infective situations

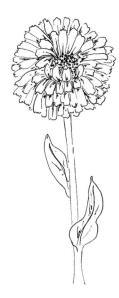

Marigold

externally. Calendula (part of the Latin name) cream is exceptionally good for cracked heels, rain scald and other skin infections. It can be purchased easily and can also make a very good handcream for human hands that suffer from too much stable work in the winter!

CHAMOMILE
Chamomile tea is very useful for horses and humans with competition nerves. The dried herb can be fed to nervous individuals especially those prone to 'nervous' colic. The fresh herb should not be used since it can cause mouth ulcers.

COMFREY
A herb which has caused a great deal of controversy. Since the active ingredient (allantoin) can be absorbed through the skin, the safest advice is only to use an external cream or ointment in cases of

minor fractures and other minor damage. However, it is important not to use this cream on any wound which may still be dirty. Comfrey accelerates healing and dirt may be trapped inside the wound. Comfrey has also been implicated in cases of proudflesh. Having said all this many owners swear by comfrey for healing of bone and joint problems and comfrey is readily available in dried form and easily grown in the garden. The choice is with the individual owner.

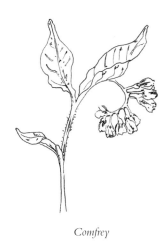

Comfrey

KELP

This is usually known as seaweed. It is a plant rich in minerals, especially calcium, iodine and potassium. For this reason it promotes hoof and coat growth and is much used by show exhibitors to ensure a sleek and shiny coat. Seaweed is at risk of contamination from heavy metals and therefore is best purchased as a dried powder especially designed for feeding to horses.

FENUGREEK

This has been widely used since ancient times for everything from treating bronchitis to fattening up women in some patrs of the world so they commanded a larger dowry when they married. For horses it is very valuable as a tonic and appetiser. Although the powder smells strongly of curry, horses seem to really enjoy the taste and it will often tempt a fussy feeder. It can also improve the flow of milk in nursing mothers, but should be avoided during pregnancy. Fenugreek is ideal for putting condition on show horses, especially those who are difficult to keep sufficient weight on. It will however take several weeks, if not months, to show any effect.

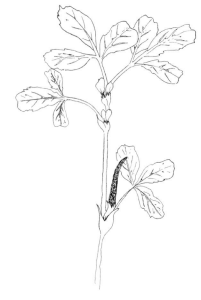

Fenugreek

How much to feed

It is important to stick to a regular routine for feeding and to remember that the more feeds you can divide the daily amount into the better. You should certainly divide your pony's ration into at least two feeds. Feed bowls or mangers should be kept clean and a different one should be kept for each pony.

There is a whole science devoted to animal feeding whereby food requirements are scientifically calculated and then rigidly adhered to. This is not really practicable for the individual owner. Basically the most important thing to do is to know how your pony should look in ideal condition and then keep him that way by minor adjustments to his feed until you obtain a balance. Horses are condition scored by the amount of flesh that they have over their hipbones. The table goes like this:

CONDITION SCORES

- 0 – starvation; bones prominent.

- 1 – thin; bones prominent but some flesh.

- 2 – approaching normal; hips bones defined but not prominent (as seen in fit horses).

- 3 – getting fat; bones becoming difficult to feel (show horses).

- 4 – obese; native ponies with laminitis!

It is also very important to match the amount fed to the amount of work being done. For young stock and breeding stock there should be increased food, together with a special supplement if complete food designed for the particular category is not being fed. For ponies competing in, for example, show jumping or working hunter pony there will need to be an increase in food. Ponies hunting regularly will need more. However a pony out to grass in the summer will soon be in trouble if he is also getting extra food. Indeed he may need his grazing restricted in any case. Most native ponies absolutely adore hard food, so you must harden your heart and never over feed him just because he loves it so much. It is possible to work out your pony's weight by using a weight tape and making calculations. You can do this when he is at the weight you think is ideal and then do it again periodically to ensure that you are keeping him to roughly the same weight.

There is a simple but effective table which tells you the ratio of concentrates to hay that you should be feeding according to various work levels:

FEEDING GUIDELINES

- Resting   – no work at all (but not breeding stock)   = hay 100 per cent.
- Light work   – child's pony or elderly pony doing no work = hay 75 per cent/ concentrates 25 per cent.
- Medium work – light showing or hacking   = hay 50 per cent/ concentrates 50 per cent.
- Heavy work   – competing   = hay 25 per cent/concentrates 75 per cent.

These are not hard and fast figures by any means, but a guideline to where your feeding regime should be at as your horse gets fitter or does more work.

Each manufacturer gives guideline amounts for feeding of their product on the bag. If you are inexperienced at feeding ponies then this would be a very useful way for you to feed initially. Start with the manufacturer's recommended amount and adjust according to the needs of the individual pony.

Excitable ponies

It can sometimes be very hard to keep weight on an excitable pony. If you want to show him – especially if he is a ridden native – this can be doubly hard. Go for as much time in the field as possible coupled with plenty of slow work. Feed him one of the complete non-heating mixes and do try several different ones as different brands suit different ponies. Try also using a herbal calming supplement. These can be very effective.

EXCESS WEIGHT

Native ponies run to fat so very easily. Having been designed to live on virtually nothing they will fatten up almost overnight on good grass alone. If you have a fat pony you must act quickly to avoid laminitis with its possible long-term consequences of hoof problems, possible re-occurrences and other problems. It is important that the pony does some work at least. If he is not ridden then put him into an all-weather menage or a tiny bare paddock so that he gets some exercise by moving around. This applies too if he has laminitis. He must keep his circulation going. If he is ridden then his workload must go up gradually until he is being ridden as often as is humanely possible.

Food is a difficult problem especially where poor hoof condition might be or has become

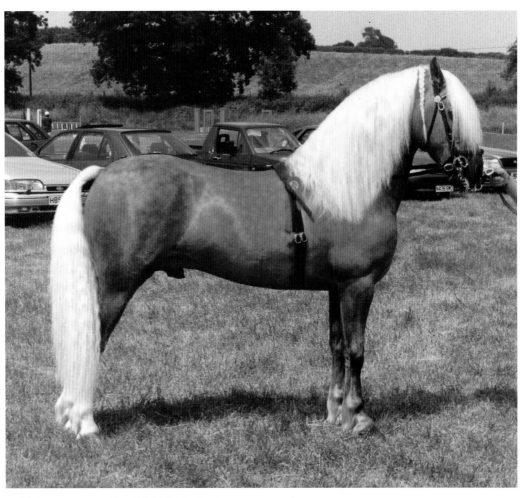

Welsh Section D stallion Houndsfield Golden Brenin

a problem. It is best to feed a good supplement to avoid any vitamin or mineral deficiency and to put it into a feed of dampened bran with some carrots or apples. Usually if a pony has become grossly fat he will be greedy anyway so will eat this readily.

You must also keep his intake of fibre up. The best way to do this is with some very soft, poor quality (but not musty or dusty) meadow hay. He should have his hay ration divided into as many portions as is practicable so that his gut is kept occupied as much of the time as possible. If you feed him his ration all at once he will eat it in a very short time and then will not have anything in his gut for the rest of the twenty-four hours which can lead to colic and other digestive disorders.

Remember that you are looking to decrease his calorie intake in proportion to the amount of work he does just as you need to if you need to lose weight yourself. However, just as in humans, starvation is never the answer. It can only lead to deficiencies and other problems.

RULES OF GOOD FEEDING

• Water should be available at all times except after strenuous exercise. If the pony has not had water available for any reason, offer it before feeding.

• Never feed when hot or tired from exercise – wait at least an hour.

• Never ride immediately after feeding

• Feed at regular times.

• Do not change food suddenly – this applies to hay as well as concentrates. Make the changeover gradually.

• Feed according to the condition of the pony; the work done and the amount of grass available.

• Never feed dusty, musty or mouldy forage.

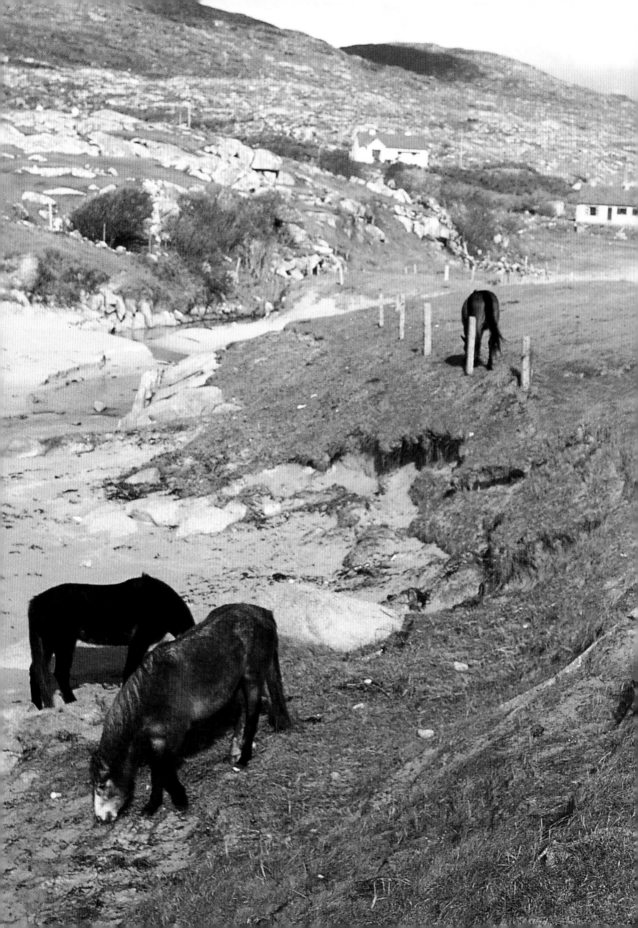

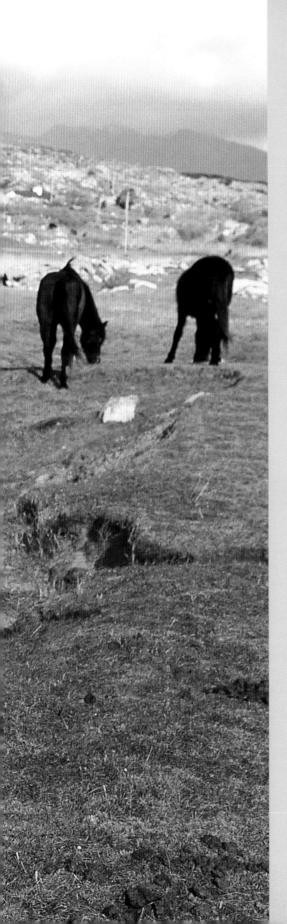

4

Promoting Good Health

How do you know if your native pony is in good health? Watch him closely. At rest he should be breathing evenly at eight to twelve breaths per minute. He should be generally relaxed, standing evenly on all four feet. The exception to this is when he rests a hind leg occasionally, putting the point of the toe to the ground. His coat should be glossy. In the summer this is easy to see but in the winter it may not be quite so noticeable. In winter, however, his coat should stand out evenly from his body and feel soft and dry. Grease will come off it when brushed or stroked with the hand but the coat should not *look* greasy.

His mane and tail may well be very full and bushy or may be thinner than this but any unexplained bald patches should be subject to further investigation. His legs should be free from previously unnoticed lumps and bumps and his hooves should be slightly glossy (under the coating of mud) and not showing signs of cracking or splitting. His heels should be clean and dry with no signs of skin irritation. Make a

Connemara Ponies in their natural enviroment 67

habit of feeling your pony's legs each time you pick out his hooves. You will soon get to know what is normal for him and will immediately notice anything unusual.

His eyes should be clear and bright and in the case of a native pony usually have a twinkle! There should be no sign of discharge or stickiness and he should be able to open them both fully. His nostrils should be clean and slightly damp. Again there should be no sign of discharge or redness. Breathing with flared nostrils and a raised breathing rate can be a sign of a raised temperature. Native ponies' ears are hardly ever still. They can be held right forward, indicating anticipation or curiosity at something new. They can be held at rest, neither forward nor back, but tending towards forward. They can prick backwards and forwards which means his brain is working. The only position that is not so good is back. Just holding them back can indicate stress or other unhappiness such as pain. This position can show a dislike of a person, another horse or a procedure such as rugging up. If he stands looking miserable with his ears back and no real reason for this you must investigate further and check for other signs of disease or injury. If he puts his ears back flat against his head, watch you do not get bitten!

When you put him out in the field or if you call him over to you he should move freely using all four legs equally. Lameness can be difficult for the inexperienced person to detect, but again if you know your own pony well you will almost sense something is wrong even if it is difficult to see. His head should be carried neither too high nor too low, and not held to one side.

His tail should be carried according to the breed standard. For example the Welsh carry their tail much more 'gaily' than say a Shetland, but no pony should have his tail clamped down except during very wet and/or cold weather.

As he moves his breathing should be free from any kind of noise, especially rasping which could either indicate infection or allergic problems. He might be puffing if he is unfit; this is normal.

In freezing conditions or in snow there are some other considerations which should be observed to keep your pony healthy. Firstly he must always have access to unfrozen water. Dehydrated animals stop moving around and soon add cold to their other problems. You should also look carefully at his coat. It is quite all right for him to have icicles in his mane and tail and probably on his eyelashes. This will not hurt. However, the vet who was called out to a very lame pony one snowy day was surprised to find that the pony's damp tail had frozen to his damp leg as he stood sheltering during the worst of the night. When the temperature failed to rise in the morning the tail remained firmly affixed to the leg and the pony could hardly move! Ponies, even native ponies, require feeding during bad weather. Please consult chapter three for further advice.

Droppings are a very good indicator of health. They vary according to the diet being currently fed. For the stable-kept pony in the winter, whose main bulk of food is hay the droppings will be light brown in colour and slightly damp and fibrous in texture, each ball breaking slightly when hitting the ground. They would normally be passed around eight times a day with no straining or difficulty. A pony at grass in the summer would have droppings much greener in colour. They could well be slightly wetter than the stabled pony but should not be liquid or foul smelling. Urine is passed several times a day and is pale yellow when a normal colour. A pony assumes a straddling position to pass urine. The back legs are put further back and out to the sides and the tail is held out. Whilst this looks uncomfortable, a view that may be further reinforced by the groaning that some ponies do, it is normal. What is not normal is straddling but not passing any urine; passing urine that is very dark or foul smelling and passing urine with blood in it.

Taking your pony's temperature

You should take the pony's temperature if you suspect that he may be ill. This will be useful information for the vet when you call him. Use a proper animal thermometer which is more robust than one designed for human use. A human one can be used in an emergency with care. First tie the pony up or have him held by an assistant. Shake down the mercury until it is below 37.4°C (99.3°F). Grease the bulb end with Vaseline. Lift the tail and insert about two thirds of it for thirty seconds. Be certain to grip the thermometer very firmly. The action of the bowel can sometimes draw it in unexpectedly. Retrieve the thermometer and check. The normal temperature should be 38°C (100.4°F). It can go up in

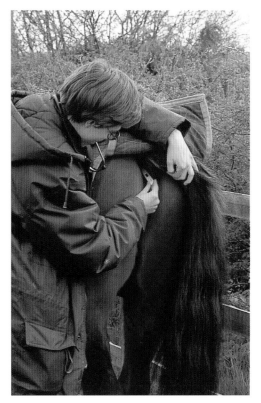

Taking a pony's temperature

warm weather, after exercise, and some ponies do have a slightly higher temperature as their normal level.

Taking your pony's pulse

The pulse can be found in several places. One of the easiest is on the face, just underneath the top of the lower jaw. If you watch carefully you will see the facial artery beating in that area and will know just where to put your fingers. There is another place on the face, just above and behind the eye, in an area roughly corresponding to your own temple. The third place is on the leg, which may be difficult with a hairy

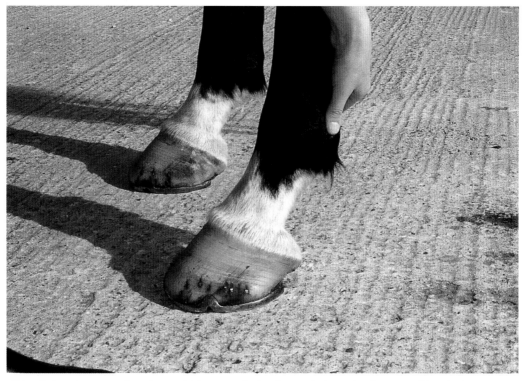

Although the pulse is most often taken on the face it can also be taken on the leg as this illustration of digital pulse measurement shows

pony, but is on the inside of the front knee. The normal pulse should be between thirty-six and forty-two beats per minute. Take your pony's pulse when he is well and at rest, so that you will know exactly how to do it if you suspect he is unwell. A raised pulse rate, just like a raised temperature, is a sign that all is not well.

By having a native pony you are at least half way towards having a healthy animal. In-built hardiness and resistance to climate and conditions have genetically given us a pretty tough animal. However, we have to remember that this does not mean that we can neglect basic health care, especially when you remember that most of our native ponies are now kept in artificial conditions. This is coupled with the fact that in the last fifty years or so some ponies have been bred for show winning qualities rather than pure native grit.

The foot and shoeing

I am sure you will have heard the old saying 'no foot, no horse,' but just think about it in more depth. The whole of your pony's weight is carried on four feet each measuring only a few inches across. The foot is composed of bones, namely part of the second phalanx, the third phalanx (coffin bone) and sesamoid of the third phalanx (navicular bone). At each side of the coffin bone are two plates of cartilages. They are often referred to as side bones if ossification has resulted from various conditions. Covering the bones of the foot are sensitive tissues. These are technically called the prododermic tissues and are similar in composition to skin, having a good supply both of blood vessels and nerves. These tissues are also referred to as the laminae, and are the origin of the name of the condition laminitis.

We all know the part of the foot that we can see – the hoof wall. It is a protective coating for the more vulnerable parts of the foot. It is in effect very much the same as our own finger nails – a kind of modified and hardened skin. The sole of the foot is the part which you clean with a hoof pick and is crescent shaped. It protects the coffin bone. At the back of the sole is the frog. This is a sensitive triangular piece of elastic tissue which acts as a cushion for the foot.

Most small native ponies, especially Shetland, Dartmoor, Exmoor and Welsh Section A, can spend their whole lives without shoes as long as their feet are regularly trimmed and well maintained by a good farrier. The only reason for shoes for such a pony is in cases of foot problems where corrective shoeing is required or if the pony has to do great amounts of road work, for example in the case of a driving pony.

Daily maintenance of the feet must include regular picking out and inspection of the foot. Care should be taken to notice anything different about the foot, for example if the pony flinches when a certain area is scraped with the hoof pick. This may indicate that a foreign body has infiltrated the foot and an infection is developing. Cracks which appear and run vertically up the hoof or down from the coronet band should be attended to without delay. They will need the attention of the farrier. Any foul smell from the foot, especially the frog, could indicate a fungal infection. The foot should be thoroughly scrubbed with a salt water solution and the area sprayed with purple spray or a proprietary product. If the problem persists more than a few days you should consult your vet. Any sign of discharge at the coronet band or elsewhere is a matter for the vet also.

The healthy foot does not really need hoof oil, although it can be applied to very dry brittle feet to help them and of course no horse is properly dressed without it in the show ring.

SHOEING

If your pony needs shoes then you will need to visit the farrier or have him visit you every six weeks. You will need to ensure that your pony has had practise in having his feet handled and will stand quietly. You should provide a firm surface, with good lighting in the winter. The pony should be ready with his legs and feet clean at the appointed time. Farriers have developed a very bad reputation for turning up hours (or even days!) late. If your farrier does this get another one. The Farriers Registration Council (see address list) supplies a free list.

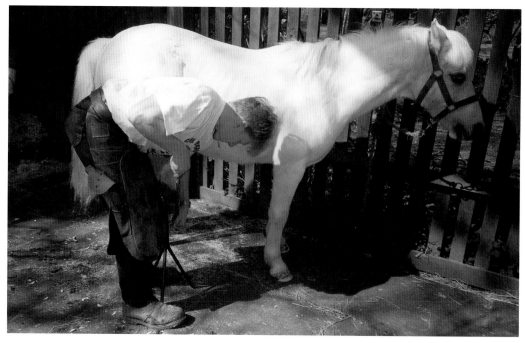

Regular visits from the farrier are very important even after a pony is retired

The picture of good health – Supreme Ridden Champion Aston True Welshman ridden by Emma Bexson

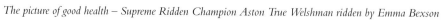

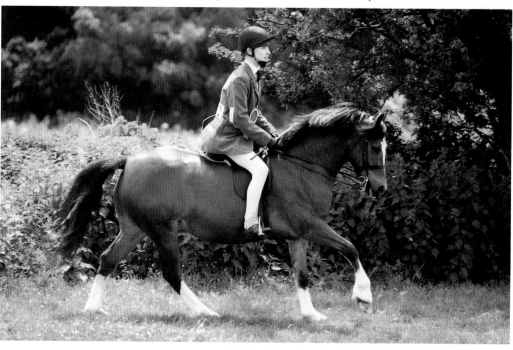

THE WELL-SHOD FOOT

It is important that you familiarise yourself with what a well-shod foot should look like. There is a free leaflet published by the Worshipful Company of Farriers (available from the F.R.C.) which gives a good idea. The main points are as follows:

• The shoe should be of the correct weight and size for the pony and for the job he is doing.

• It should fit the foot exactly, with no gaps anywhere and no places where the shoe overlaps the edge of the foot or vice-versa.

• The clenches should be in a neat line, not too far up the hoof or too near the shoe and not protruding out.

• Your pony should be completely sound from the moment the work is done. If there is any sign of lameness call the farrier back at once. He is required by law to attend as soon as possible in these circumstances.

A good farrier is a mine of useful advice about foot care and shoeing. He will advise the best shoes for your pony and in a long-term relationship he will note problems with your pony, probably long before you do. For example, he may well note the first signs of laminitis.

When to call the vet

We all know that veterinary treatment is relatively expensive – a good incentive to keep your pony as healthy as you possibly can. However, sometimes, despite our best efforts he will need expert help. There are several matters which would require urgent attention:

WHEN TO CALL THE VET

• A temperature raised above 39°C (102.2°F).

• Heavy or laboured breathing which is not the result of strenuous exercise.

• Any wound from which the bleeding cannot be controlled or any wound which will require stitching.

• A pony showing signs of pain such as standing, possibly hunched and showing reluctance to move.

• A pony showing signs of colic. This may be a general restlessness possibly with an increase in the rate of breathing. He may look at his flanks and may get up and down and try to roll. Colic can progress very quickly and always needs the vet if it does not subside very quickly.

Always ensure that the pony is either stabled or confined in a shelter before the vet arrives. It can be difficult for a vet to examine a pony in the middle of a field in a howling blizzard. Anyone keeping ponies even if they do keep them out all the year round should really have a stable available for emergencies. At night or during the winter, provision of at least some light will also be helpful. The vet will want to wash his hands after he has examined the pony. If you have any doubt about remembering his instructions have a notebook and pen ready to take notes. When you are distressed by your pony's illness or accident it can sometimes be very difficult to remember instructions and they are of the utmost importance.

Worms and worming

All horses carry worms and if not kept under control, they can seriously affect the health of the animal. There are a number of different worms which affect the horse but the most common are:

ROUNDWORMS (ASCARIDS)
These develop in the liver and lungs and then the small intestine. Paddocks grazed regularly by stock often have a heavy contamination. Older horses seem to develop immunity and if not grazing with mares and foals should not be too greatly affected.

REDWORM (LARGE STRONGYLES)
Redworm develops in the intestines and is the most common parasite in horses kept in very poor conditions. It can ultimately cause death.

BOT (*GASTEROPHILUS* SPECIES)
This develops in the stomach. The eggs are laid on the horse's legs and shoulders during the summer; the horse then licks them off and ingests them. Any tiny yellowish eggs that are spotted on the coat should be removed immediately by scraping off with a razor.

THREADWORM (*STRONGYLOIDES WESTEREI*)
Most commonly affects foals and can be passed from the mare via her milk. Mares should be treated regularly to lessen the risk and foals routinely wormed at a week old.

PINWORM (*OXYURIS EQUI*)
An intestinal parasite usually kept well under control by routine worming.

LUNGWORM (*DICTYOCAULUS ARNFIELDI*)
As the name suggests this parasite infests the lungs, causing coughing. Myth says that horses and donkeys should not be kept together because horses being kept with donkeys inevitably catch this parasite. The truth is that many donkeys do carry lungworm but do not seem to be affected by it. If you keep a donkey and a pony together then routinely worm them both and there will be no problem.

TAPEWORM (*ANOPLOCEPHALA PERFOLIATA*)
This develops in the intestines and can cause problems in the area where the small and large intestines join. It is often the cause of worm related colics and other

digestive disturbances. Forage mites are part of the life cycle of this parasite. It is not the easiest parasite to treat effectively, so if you believe your pony has this then you must use a wormer especially for the problem.

All ponies should be wormed every four to six weeks, especially if they live in a place where there are other equines. Whilst one pony living alone and where grazing rotation is possible might in theory only need worming occasionally, it is always better to be safe than sorry. Products should be chosen according to the time of year and the perceived problem. For example if you buy a new pony always use a product which includes redworm treatment. A wormer including bot treatment should be used in the spring and autumn. Every saddler or pet shop selling horse wormers must by law have someone on the premises who has undergone a proper training course and can advise as to the correct product to buy if you have any doubts.

If you suspect a horse has a serious worm burden then he should be confined to the stable for forty-eight hours whilst being treated. Your vet can do a worm count from a dung sample and a blood test if you are really worried.

Remember too that worms live for various amounts of time on pasture. Good pasture management – either regular harrowing or collecting droppings if this is feasible will do much to reduce the number of worms and therefore the potential infestation level.

Alternative medicine

Horse owners are increasingly turning to alternative medicine to keep their animals healthy. The best known are:

• Homoeopathy
• Chiropractic
• Acupuncture
• Massage
• Herbal Medicine

There are many other treatments such as magnet therapy, aromatherapy and healing to name just a few. Most have strong anecdotal evidence to support their use but no real scientific basis for their claims. Horse owners with chronic problems with their animals may be tempted to try one or several of these therapies. Nothing can be lost (except presumably money!) and much could be gained. However it is possibly best to try the well-accepted methods first.

HOMOEOPATHY

This is practised in much the same way as on humans and is administered by a vet who is also a registered homoeopath. However there are some remedies which can be tried safely by the amateur. Homoeopathic tablets can be given in the 6c strength or if available in 30c strength to horses. Tablets are usually sold in 6c strength in chemist shops for human use. Occasionally 30c strength is available but as a general rule this strength would only be available in saddlers and other outlets which supply equine homoeopathic products or from a homoeopathic vet.

They should be given twice a day and can either be tipped into the mouth or fed in a small piece of food.

Arnica

This is the sovereign remedy for bruising (both for humans and for horses). It can be given as tablets and is also usefully available in cream and ointment, designed for human use but equally effective for horses.

Rhus tox

This is the remedy for aches and pains especially those which become chronic such as arthritis.

Apis mel

For insect bites and other conditions with itching and or fluid swelling such as windgalls.

Graphites

For conditions where the skin is damaged but not by a wound. This could include mud fever and sweet itch.

There are a number of other remedies, which can be very useful for horses, but expert advice should be sought before administration.

CHIROPRACTIC

Chiropractic is a hands-on technique for re-alignment of the skeleton. It needs to be carried out by a qualified practitioner who will have first had to qualify in human chiropractic before going on to qualify to treat animals. It can be quite expensive, but does produce some spectacular results.

ACUPUNCTURE

This works in exactly the same way in horses as it does in humans and can have very good results when administered by a skilled practitioner. There are some claims that acupuncture cures vices such as crib-biting and box walking and it may be that the treatment relaxes the animal and balances him so that stress is not such a factor in his life. Increasing evidence is available which shows that there is a genetic predisposition to these vices so that it can be worth a try as long as you do not expect miracles.

MASSAGE

Massage is definitely the latest 'in' therapy. Competition horses travel to events with their own masseur much the same as human athletes. You can learn to massage your horses yourself in a general way but specific problems are best left to a qualified person. Massage can also have huge benefits in conditions such as laminitis whereby the muscles are tensed continually with the pain in the feet, causing muscle spasms to appear in other places. Massage really relieves these problems.

HERBAL MEDICINE

Some herbs are included in the feeding chapter, if they are suitable to use as a feed supplement for various conditions. Other herbs which can be useful for horses are listed below. Herbs can be used with any other therapy and can usually be used alongside conventional drugs to support the rest of the body whilst the injured part is treated with antibiotics or whatever.

Red clover

A head of clover flowers can be a very useful first aid for insect bites (both for the pony and for you). They can also be used either raw or made into an infusion for irritating skin conditions such as sweet itch.

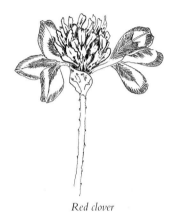

Red clover

Rosehips

Rosehips are considered to have use in laminitis. They certainly contain biotin which is thought to help hoof growth and are used in Chinese herbal medicine as a liver tonic – which all laminitics need. Gather the hips in the autumn and remove the seeds wearing rubber gloves. Then mince and dry the flesh.

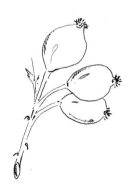

Rosehip

Raspberry

Raspberry leaves are useful for all pregnant mares during the last few weeks of pregnancy and whilst feeding the foal. They tone up the uterine muscles and enhance milk flow. Do not use in early pregnancy.

Coltsfoot

This herb is very good for dry coughs and for easing the breathing of ponies with long term COPD. You can buy the syrup for human use and either put it into the horse's mouth with a syringe or put it on some apple on top of the feed.

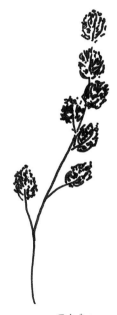

Coltsfoot

Devil's claw

This herb has long been used for human aches and pains especially arthritis. It is now increasingly available in preparations for equine use. Do not use during pregnancy.

Valerian

The great calmer. This can also be used for competition nerves and for horses getting nervous colic when travelling or competing. Buy a preparation intended for equine use and never exceed the stated dose. Giving more will not make the horse calmer and can cause unwanted side effects. Do not use regularly.

St John's wort

Use as a cream for wound healing. This herb encourages granulation and may cause 'proudflesh' if used to excess.

Witch hazel

A useful item for the first aid chest. A dilution can be used to bathe eyes and to cold compress bruising.

Common injuries and illnesses

WOUNDS

Every pony gets wounds at some time or other. They can range from the scrapes and grazes which come from skirmishes in the field to serious wounds arising from accidents. The first action is to clean the wound unless it is very serious in which case the vet should be called urgently. Bleeding should stop very quickly, if it does not pressure should be applied to the wound with a clean pad whilst waiting for the vet to arrive.

For less serious wounds wash off any dirt and assess the situation. Puncture wounds are quite common in ponies who get thorns in their coat whilst foraging in the hedge. These should be watched carefully for swelling which indicates festering and may mean a foreign body is still inside the wound. Poultice this type of wound and get veterinary advice if the pony shows signs of illness or the wound does not clear up quickly.

Other wounds which do not require veterinary attention should be kept clean at all times and treated with a proprietary wound powder. Covering is not necessary for small wounds. Remember to keep up your pony's tetanus protection.

LAMENESS

Lameness can occur in the pony for a myriad of reasons. Trot him up and down on a hard surface to discern the affected leg. If both front legs are affected it may well be laminitis (*qv*). For a single leg, when you have discovered which one it is, you should check down the leg carefully for swelling and pick out the hoof thoroughly in case of a trapped stone. Even a tiny stone can make some ponies very lame. If he is shod check the shoe for looseness or raised clenches. Seek veterinary advice if the cause of your pony's lameness is not immediately obvious and does not clear up within a day or so. Sometimes ponies can pull a muscle and this will clear itself very quickly when the pony walks about in the field. Indeed unless the lameness is very severe the best first course of action can be to put him in the field and see if things right themselves.

FEVERS, COUGHS AND COLDS

These usually start with the pony just looking generally off colour. He may refuse his feed or just stand looking miserable. Shivering and an increase in breathing are often the next symptoms. This is the time to take his temperature. For a raised temperature you should call the vet immediately. Isolate the pony if possible in case the problem is contagious. Keep him warm.

The vet will usually prescribe antibiotics, but there is much you can do to speed his recovery. Garlic is a great natural antibiotic. Try to get him to eat fresh crushed cloves if you can; up to five a day. Keep his nose clean and burn the cotton wool that you use. Keep him warm but put him in the field for a short time if the weather is warm and sunny. Pick green food (but never feed grass cuttings) for him if he cannot go out. This should include dandelions if you can find them. Follow your vet's instructions carefully.

COLIC

Colic is used to describe abdominal pain and can vary from a vague grumbling in the tummy of a pony who has found fallen apples in the field to the very serious symptoms of twisted gut. The best rule to follow is to confine the pony in the stable at the first sign of symptoms and to call the vet if they have not started to improve after twenty minutes. Obviously, if you do not find him until symptoms are clearly giving him great distress then call the vet immediately making it clear that it is a colic and that you require an urgent visit. You will know a serious colic if you see one and no amount of words will describe the distress it will cause both you and the pony. Thankfully however most colics are easily resolved.

LAMINITIS

Laminitis is the scourge of every native pony. Having evolved to live on next to nothing he is suddenly put into a rich green lowland field and allowed to stuff himself silly. Laminitis can be 'encouraged' by other factors such as too much work on hard ground. However the fundamental starting point is one of excessive feeding in relation to work.

If the liver – and the horse's liver is very important – cannot cope with the carbohydrate load imposed on it, the body almost panics. The temperature rises and the pulse rate increases. This means that blood flow to the foot is increased. The inside tissues of the foot swell and press against the hard outer casing of the hoof. The result is pain and the characteristic stance of a pony with laminitis. He will stand back on his heels, trying very hard to take some of the weight off his painful soles. If only the front feet are affected he may stand resting a front foot. All this means that if your pony has a raised temperature and unexplained lameness then you should suspect laminitis and call your vet. Sometimes you can see the facial pulse racing and almost always feel the digital pulse pounding away.

The most important first aid is to get the pony off the grass and into a stable or other confined area with a good thick quantity of bedding. The feet can be cold hosed to help with the pain. Your vet will prescribe a regime of treatment and medication and it has to be said that every vet has their own favourite combination of treatments and you should follow their advice.

However, there is much that you can do

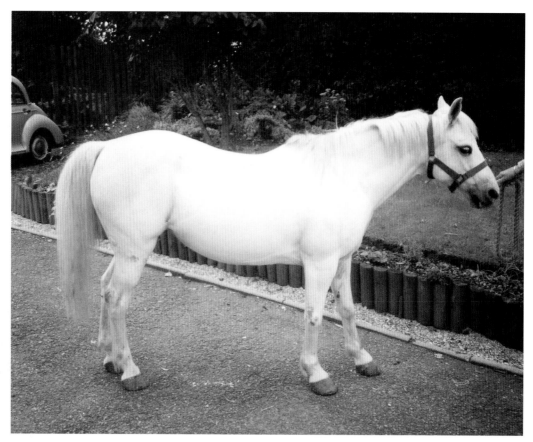

Typical laminitic stance. Note the overlong feet which are not helping this pony

The damaged feet of a pony with chronic laminitis

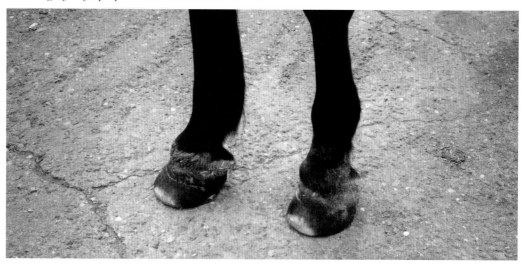

for your pony to support his recovery without interfering with veterinary treatment. If you have access to a menage or all weather surface then this is where your pony should live. He can move about exactly as much or as little as he chooses and all movement will help to keep his circulation going. Cold hose his feet at least twice a day. It is not a cure but it really does seem to help. If you have a stream stand him in it when he is well enough to walk there.

A very vital part of the recovery programme is correct foot trimming. For this you really need a specialist farrier who is able to do veterinary remedial work – not all qualified farriers can do this. It is expensive but very important to your pony's recovery. Shoes are usually removed from shod ponies to begin with and should only be replaced when the vet advises. Sadly laminitis very often causes the sole of the foot to drop which may mean special shoeing. The dropped sole is a result of pedal bone rotation. Occasionally, the pedal bone can rotate so much that it protrudes through the sole of the foot. This only occurs after prolonged suffering with this disease and indicates the need for swift action as soon as you have any suspicion of laminitis at all. If the pedal bone protrudes then the pony almost inevitably has to be destroyed.

Whilst nursing your pony you will not be able to put him out in a field. It can be useful therefore to give him some green food – just enough to keep him happy. This food is increased in value if it contains useful herbs to aid his recovery. Dandelions are the first choice. As a diuretic and liver tonic they are ideal for him. Sow thistle has similar properties. Cleavers (goose grass) is useful too but is not always eaten. Pot Marigolds (not the garden variety but *Calendula officinalis*) are useful too, having anti-inflammatory action. Feed just the petals. Last but not least is the ever useful garlic. Try to get him to eat fresh cloves (possibly inserted into a slice of apple) and go for five or six cloves a day if you can.

Once a pony has had laminitis he seems to get a pre-disposition to further attacks. Keep him on restricted grazing. Fence part of your field off if necessary. Do not think that you can just put him out for an hour on lush grazing and keep him in the rest of the time. The gorging he can do in that time will almost certainly cause problems. He is better out all the time on a paddock with no grass on. However, do remember that the paddock might look bare and the pony might still be eating too much. By his constant eating he is keeping the grass from appearing to grow! Be very vigilant and you should be able to keep him going for many years.

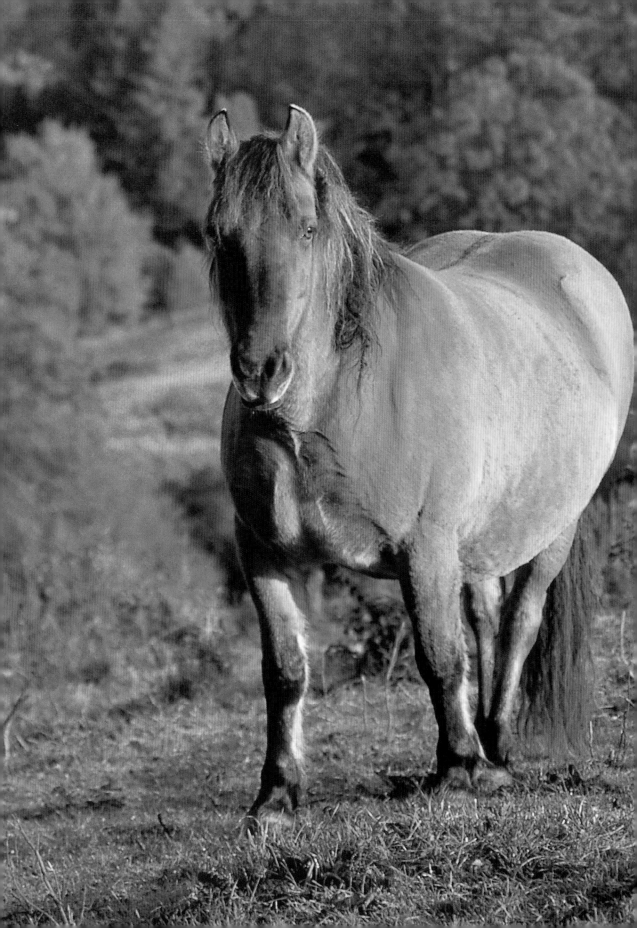

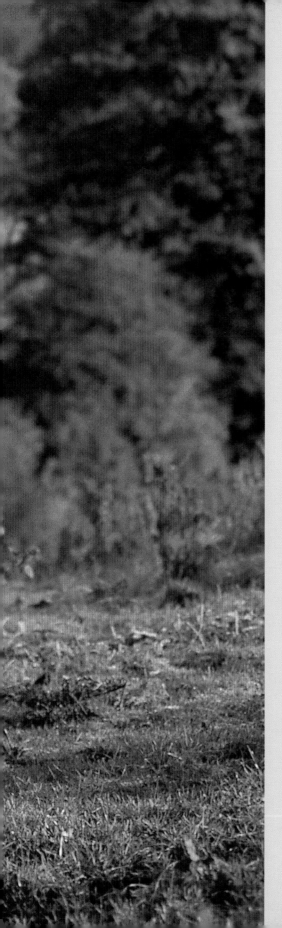

5

Grooming and Coat Care

Coat

The native pony, by the very virtue of his natural habitat, has a thick coat in the winter. For the owner who keeps ponies for breeding and wants them to live out in the winter, it is a godsend. For those people who want to ride their pony (and those who want to show at early shows) much can be done to temper the natural inclination to woolliness.

For the pony who is going to be kept out and not ridden, the very barest of attention is required. Too much grooming will deplete the coat of natural oils, which are there to protect against wet weather. This is why it is always better not to use a New Zealand rug unless you have to. The rug will 'rub off' the coat oils and flatten the coat down. A coat which has not been flattened by a rug will be full of tiny air bubbles which also add to insulation.

It is important, however, just to feel over the coat thoroughly every so often and to remove bits of twig and thorns which may pierce the skin. This is a good opportunity to feel for lumps and bumps or other problems which may have arisen and may be hidden by a thick coat. The tail should be kept short enough so that it does not drag on the ground. There have been cases of ponies standing sheltering on a freezing night and actually having their tail frozen to the grass where they stood. However, do not under any circumstances thin the tip of the tail or shorten the mane in any way. These are nature's way of protecting the pony. If you feel underneath the thick mane of a native pony on a cold day, it is as good as warming your hands by a fire.

If you want a short coat for winter riding or for early in-hand shows, then you must start rugging up in August. See the section on page 96 for further details.

The clipped coat will be very easy to care for. If your pony is kept in and rugged up at night then you can use as much grooming as you want to keep his coat in good condition. There is no need to worry about stripping essential oils. If you bath him, he will dry off more quickly.

The summer coat on most native ponies is the complete opposite to their winter coat. It is often short and silky and unless the pony is ill or malnourished it should gleam with health. If your native pony is less than twenty years old and has a dull summer coat then you should get your vet to check him over. Even if he is not showing any sign of illness, a dull coat is unusual and you may catch some serious illness before it develops by using this indicator. The winter coat can be dull for no reason other than an accumulation of dust and dirt.

In summer it is very important to give thought to any white areas your pony might have. Global warming and ozone layer holes have made the sun more risky for us all – including ponies. White marking on the face, especially where there is pink skin should be covered with (human) sun block every day to avoid burning. White legs are usually all right apart from the heels which should also be treated with sunblock. A pony with very pink skin is often best kept inside during the day and put out at night in hot and sunny weather.

There are some very good supplements on the market for improving the coat. These are especially beneficial if you have recently purchased a pony which has been in poor bodily condition and also to boost coat shine in others. The very best and cheapest supplement is the herb fenugreek. Many of the feed manufacturers are now selling it as a powder. It will make your stables smell of curry but it is an excellent conditioner and is good value for money. It is also useful for putting weight on without increasing excitability.

Certain of the societies have rules which apply specifically to the coat. The Welsh Pony and Cob Society is a good example of this. They say that 'animals, three years old and under cannot be clipped for showing purposes. Animals four years old and over, which have been clipped for winter activities can be shown at early spring shows with their coats growing back – no fresh clipping'.

Since all the breed societies have different rules and they do change them from time to time, you should check up on the latest rules before you get the clippers out!

The same advice applies to trimming below the jawline and around the ears. If you do trim the jaw, for example on a Welsh Section B, you should make the job look as natural as possible. I have yet to see anyone achieve a natural look with clippers, unless they are very skilled. For the amateur it is always better to use the scissors and to brush the hair down again between 'cuts' so that you are sure you are keeping a natural line. To avoid 'stepping' in the hair you should always brush the coat up in the opposite way to its natural lie and cut with the scissors lying against the skin with the points going in the opposite way to the coat. For example if you are cutting off excess feather you should brush the hair upwards on the leg and then hold the scissors with the points facing upwards. When you brush the hair down again the look should be reasonably natural.

Personally, I believe it is cruel to cut off the whiskers. We are not really sure of their function, but ponies who have their whiskers suddenly cut off can develop head shaking, skin rashes and other problems, which proves to me at least that they are there for a purpose and should be left in-situ.

GROOMING KIT AND HOW TO USE IT

The first thing to remember when grooming is that it is much easier when the pony is tied up! Although you might feel that it is easy to groom a stabled pony without tying him, unless he is very quiet, it will be natural for him to move around and he will end up treading on the kit box

and making you frustrated with him.

Your grooming kit should be kept together in a suitable box, and cleaned regularly. Brushes are washed in water with a little detergent and a few drops of suitable disinfectant or tea tree oil. They are best left out to dry in the sun. Although you can dry them on a radiator or similar in the winter, this will eventually damage wooden-backed brushes.

It is not a good idea to share a grooming kit or to use the same one for several ponies. It can spread infection or fungal problems such as ringworm.

Grooming is an important part of stable routine and something which almost every pony enjoys. However, it can be difficult to groom a kept-out native pony, especially if it has been raining. If this is the case and if you want to ride him, your only course of action is to dry the areas under his saddle and bridle as best you can – a cactus cloth which is usually readily available from saddlers can be very useful for this task.

If he comes in from the field dry but filthy, then your best course of action is to start with a plastic curry comb. Purists will tell you that this is an implement designed for cleaning the body brush, but quite frankly it is just about the only thing which will get off caked-on dry mud. However, be careful with it on the face and over bony

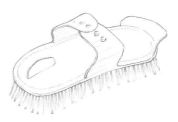

Curry comb

parts of the legs. A plastic curry comb can also be a useful tool for getting rid of surplus mane and/or tail. It pulls out a certain amount of hair during brushing and regular use will lessen the amount of hair. For this reason, obviously, you would not use it on a thin mane or tail. The rubber curry comb, also designed for cleaning the body brush, is exceptionally good for removing loose hair during moulting.

Generally speaking, the body brush, which has soft dense bristles, is used on the mane and tail and face and on the whole coat during the summer. It removes dust and grease and is used with long sweeping strokes, passing it through the curry comb

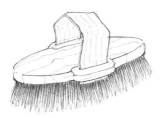

Body brush

every few strokes, to clean it. Body brushing of the main coat is a waste of time in the winter and will also remove precious insulating grease. However, body brushing in the summer is a very rewarding activity. – it brings a good gloss to the coat. The body brush is used on the mane and tail to separate out the hairs and get them hanging as neatly as is possible in a native pony. The legs are brushed gently with a dandy brush in winter. The stiffer longer bristles of a dandy brush are also often employed to remove stubborn mud patches on the summer coat and can also be used on very thick manes and tails. Longer feather can be separated out by hand

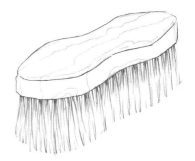

Dandy brush

before brushing if it is stuck together with mud. A final polish can be achieved with a soft cloth – an old tea towel is ideal.

You would not normally use a mane comb on a native pony – this is really only used for pulling the mane and tail and in plaiting. However, it is useful to have one in your kit, because it can be employed to get stubborn tangles or bits of stick or other debris out of the mane and tail.

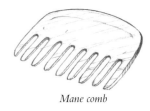

Mane comb

The eyes and nose should be cleaned with one sponge and the dock with another. These sponges should be kept separate and soaked every so often in a solution of Dettol or something similar to prevent bacterial infection.

Hooves should be picked out into a suitable receptacle. A very useful tool for use on native ponies is the hoof pick which incorporates a stiff brush. Mud covering the outer surface of the hoof needs to be removed to check for raised clenches (if shod) and to check the hoof for damage.

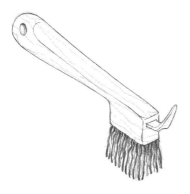

Hoof pick incorporating stiff brush

The most important consideration when grooming is to remember to ensure that the pony is as clean as possible in any area which will be covered by tack or rugs. It is very easy for a lump of mud to rub, say under the girth, and for you to end up with a girth gall (an area of skin damage often ending up raw and very painful) and not be able to ride for several weeks.

THE MANE

There can be circumstances which dictate that a mane is thinned or trimmed in the summer. For example if you have a native pony which also does Nursery Stakes under BSPS rules, then he will need to be plaited for this class. You should pull the mane as little as possible, especially if you intend to do native classes as well. You will have to practise your plaiting to get the best effect, but generally your plaits will need to be smaller and have more of them to achieve a good result. Unruly native manes respond well to being stuck into plaits with hair gel. If you need to get the plaits out for another class at the same show, then you will need lots of water. Sluice the plaits off well and then dry with a rough towel. The rubbing action will take out the kinks which will be there even if the plaits have only been in for a short while.

To get a silky mane you should use one of the proprietary mane and tail conditioners which are available everywhere. To get the mane to lie on the correct side you should plait it over, in big loose plaits when the pony is in the stable. To get a thick mane which has bits sticking up to look neat you can use either hair gel or a proprietary brand of men's hair dressing. Never be tempted to pull short bits out if they are sticking up. They will grow again and will be short bits again! It is very easy for the amateur to get bits of the mane caught in the clippers when doing a full clip or a clip which would involve removing the coat on the neck. It is a good tip to leave half an inch each side of the mane to avoid doing this and getting short ends in the spring.

If you have to tidy the mane the best way to achieve a natural look is to use a tail knife. This is a little metal comb with a razor blade attached to it. Blunt the razor blade slightly first by rubbing it on the stable wall or some other suitable object. Then take off any long ends which are obvious. If you need to shorten the mane by more than an inch or two then you can pull it, doing this carefully from underneath and continually reassessing the situation so that you do not take too much. Bear in mind that pulling also thins the mane and that the pulled hairs will grow again and will have to either be re-pulled or your pony will have to have a 'bad hair time' whilst they re-grow completely. If the mane is just too thin to pull then trim the ends with the tail knife and leave it as it is.

Do not cut a pathway for the bridle to go in – or worse still remove a portion of the mane at the withers. This looks very unnatural. You should just part the hair with your fingers or a comb when you put the bridle on. If your pony has a thin or short forelock you can often bring a portion of mane forward and give the illusion of a better forelock.

Your pony's mane is a bit like your own hair. You will learn by trial and error the best way to manage it and the best products to use to achieve that just groomed look!

TAILS

Native ponies do not have their tails pulled, nor do they have them levelled off at the bottom. Having said this, however, you will have to pull it a bit if it is very thick at the top. This should always be done from underneath and very carefully! Remember that when the tail has been pulled and washed and bandaged it will be flatter and appear thinner than when you are working on it in an unwashed state. Never, ever pull hairs from the centre even if you think they look long. They will lie down much better than short ones – trust me! To achieve a natural bottom end you should use a tail knife to shorten small sections so that the middle hairs are slightly longer than the outside ones giving a very slightly pointed effect to the finished tail.

Conditioners will allow you to work your way through a very thick tail. If you think the whole tail needs to be less, then you can use a plastic curry comb to brush it

on a daily basis. Conversely if it is too thin, never brush it unless you are going to be seen in public and then either just wash and comb gently with a wide-toothed comb or brush carefully with a soft body brush.

Gel is great for sticking down a thick tail. Spread on the gel, work it well in and then bandage just past the end of the dock. If you bandage right down you will end up with a tail that looks like a walking stick. If you have a white tail, you will have to put it into a stocking if you need to keep it clean for a show.

If your pony lives out during the winter then try to avoid washing the tail. If it is full of grease the water will just run off during rain. If there is no grease the tail will become sodden and cling to the pony's backside making him thoroughly miserable.

FEATHERS

Feathers are an integral part of the native pony's appearance. They can, however, provide all sorts of problems. The most common can be mud fever (see page 93) which leaves the legs red and sore. The best protection is the natural grease in the coat, but when legs are washed and dried for riding or whatever, this grease is lost and should be replaced either with Vaseline or some proprietary greasy potion. The legs must be absolutely dry for this to work.

Feathers should normally be left untrimmed, but this poses a problem for the pony which also competes under BSPS rules. The best compromise is to leave a small amount of feather right on the heel and to stick it down with gel for BSPS classes. It can then be 'fluffed up' for native classes and if the socks are white, thickened out with chalk or wood powder.

Feathers are a problem if you are needing to apply some form of leg protection for travelling. In fact most native ponies are so sensible that they travel perfectly happily without protection. However, if you have a long journey or are using a trailer then use thick boots. The coat can be laid down carefully before they are applied and then thickened out on arrival as best as possible. A windy day is very good for fluffing up feathers.

Clipping

Whether or not to clip is a difficult question to answer. If you intend to ride your pony in any other way than a gentle hack in the winter then you will have to clip him. You can make this look fairly natural if you are careful how you do it. The best clip for a native pony is when the coat is removed underneath the belly following a line diagonally up from the stifle to the shoulder. The neck can be given a good arch by ensuring that the line goes up slightly in the middle of the neck. The underneath of the jaw is then clipped but the front of the face is left on. This helps to keep the native look.

If you do not intend to do much work then a sweat patch can be clipped from just behind the girth, under the belly, going between the front legs and up underneath the neck and jaw.

If on the other hand you will be hunting

or showing in the winter, it is possible to clip a native pony out early, say around September or whenever his coat is growing well but is not fully through. Then you can rug him up well and the rest of his coat will grow through, leaving him with what appears to be a very fine winter coat.

The problem with clipping out is the feathers. What you have to do is to look at the legs and decide where the longer feather hairs start. These are usually arranged in an upside down 'V' shape, the 'point' being around knee level and widening out until covering the back of the fetlock. They then extend down into the heel. If you look at your pony he may well have long hairs much further up his legs, but if you include these in the clipping and just leave the areas suggested then when the coat grows again, hopefully, all will be well.

Never ever clip the feathers off altogether if you intend to show your pony. They will never grow back quite right and will have to go through an awful half grown stage on the way.

HOW TO CLIP

Decide on the pattern that you want to employ for your clip. There are the well-known ways of clipping such as a blanket clip which has just the area covered by a blanket and the legs left; a hunter clip which has just a saddle patch and the legs left and lots of others including various variations dreamed up by varying pony producers and which will identify their ponies at a glance! Clipping is very easy to learn but should be practised a bit before you clip a pony which is to appear in public. There are certain things to remember:

CLIPPING

• Always go against the lie of the coat unless you are trimming legs in which case careful use of the clippers with the lie of the coat can produce a good result.

• Always keep your clippers sharp and well oiled.

• Have at least one spare pair of blades to hand. You do not want to leave a half-clipped pony whilst you send away your blades for sharpening.

• Keep the pony warm enough both during and after clipping and whilst he gets used to his new lack of coat.

• Have an assistant to hand if you are worried about how the pony might behave. You can use a herbal tranquiliser or Bach Flowers Rescue Remedy for a pony who is slightly fidgety. It is better to get veterinary advice for a really difficult pony.

• Always use an electricity circuit breaker. These are easily obtained from DIY stores. Horses electrocute very easily and a fidgety pony can tread on and break the cable if you are not very careful. A circuit breaker stops the current immediately.

Bathing your pony

The golden rule is to get everything ready before you start. Some people bath ponies in cold water and this will do no real harm in warm weather, but quite frankly warm water is more pleasant for the pony (and for you) and will get the dirt out more easily. So you will need at least three or four buckets of warm water to start with, plus something to use for pouring the water over or you will need an appropriate hose pipe connection.

You will also need some old towels for drying the face and heels; a scraper for removing excess water; a water brush for scrubbing; a comb and your shampoo and conditioner. It is possible to buy very good horse shampoo and for ponies with problem or with very sensitive skin coats this is always best. Start with the pony's head. Use a sponge to wet the coat and shampoo only (and only a little) on stains and the forelock. You can use Johnson's baby shampoo if your pony is restless. Rinse the head and dry off before you start on the rest of the body.

You can either shampoo the whole pony and then rinse him off or wash him in sections. Obviously the first is by far the quickest but the second may be necessary in cold weather. Rinse him very thoroughly and scrape him down well. You can rub him off with old towels and should certainly dry inside the heels with an old towel. He can then be rugged up with a towelling or sweat rug and other rugs if necessary. Eating a haynet helps

Most ponies enjoy a bath including Chirk Songbird (Welsh Section B)

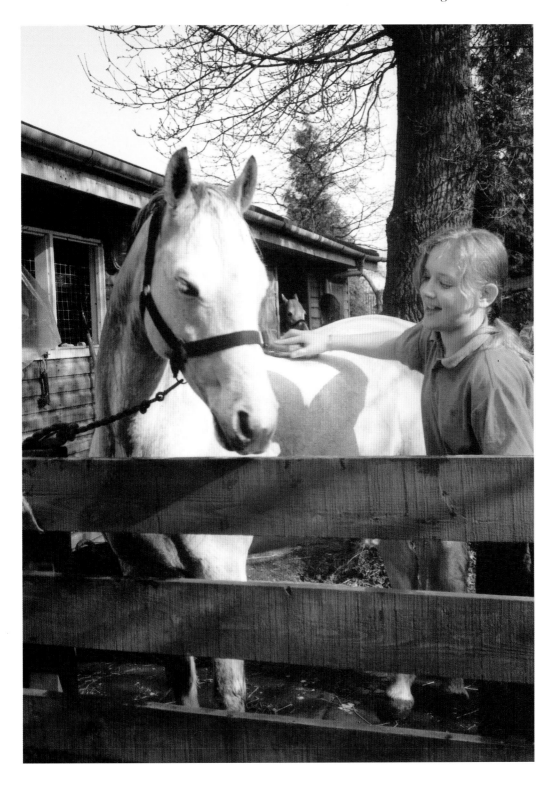

to keep him from standing entirely still and helps, therefore, to dry him. If you have heat lamps you will obviously be able to use these.

You can put a proprietary coat sheen onto his damp coat (and mane and tail) to help shine him, but this should not be done in the saddle area of ridden ponies – your saddle will slip!

The legs can be padded and bandaged if they are white legs which need to be white the next day. A good tip is to rub powdered chalk into the white legs before bandaging. When the bandages are removed the next day, the excess chalk can be brushed out of the beautifully white legs.

The mane should be combed over to the correct side and all tangles removed. If there are short ends on the top of the mane, some hair setting gel can be applied to train these down. The mane can be plaited over in loose plaits (if they are too tight the mane will be curly) or held in place by a stretch hood.

The tail should be bandaged at the top. A second bandage can be put on to cover the rest of the tail from the dock downwards or the tail can be held in a nylon stocking which is secured to the bandage. Tail hairs can be plaited for a curly effect. It is the practice of some show exhibitors to put their pony's tail in lots of small plaits to give a crinkled effect when brushed out. This is not natural but can look quite effective nevertheless. It also means that a white tail is less likely to pick up dirt overnight.

STAIN REMOVAL

The following can be very useful for stain removal on light coloured animals and on white parts.

Remember it is always better not to get the stains in the first place. This means keeping your stable very clean and removing field stains *every* day – even if it is a real chore!

STAIN REMOVAL

• Household green soap. This can be rubbed into the stain with a brush; left for a few minutes and then rinsed out thoroughly.

• Dilute hydrogen peroxide. This can be bought from the chemist and diluted in the proportions suggested for bleaching human hair. Do be careful not to use this solution on irritated skin.

• Household washing stain removal stick. This should be used sparingly and washed out thoroughly. Do not use on any area which may become irritated or on broken skin.

• Proprietary stain remover. These are very good nowadays – but also very expensive!

Coat and Hair Problems

Native ponies generally have very healthy coats and skin but there are a few problems which can affect them – mostly arising from the fact that the coat is very long!

LICE

Lice are really only found in animals in poor condition or on those which have come into contact with poor animals. They appear in the early part of the year in long coats and are usually in the mane and around the tail and rump.

The horse will be seen to rub himself on any available post or door. The treatment is to treat him with lice powder as instructed on the packet and/or to bath him thoroughly in a tea tree-based shampoo. Treatment needs to be repeated at weekly intervals to catch the nits which will have been unaffected by the first treatment and will have then hatched out.

Even though it is the worst time of year to clip a pony, if he has a bad infestation and you will be able to keep him in until his coat grows again it might be best to clip him out. Any clipping done after Christmas will affect his summer coat unless you are very lucky but if he rubs his hair off because of irritation from lice then you will not have a good coat anyway.

MUD FEVER

This is the common name for *Dermatophilus* infection and is caused by horses having wet skin for long periods of time. Standing in the field in muddy and prolonged wet weather are the kind of conditions that produce this problem. It seems to be called mud fever when it appears on the legs and rain scald when it appears on the back but both names refer to the same infection. The hair comes off in patches leaving scabby lumps which eventually come off revealing pus underneath. Treatment consists of

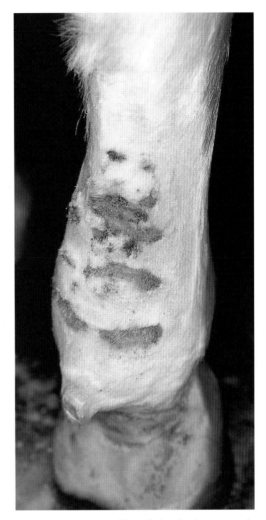

In this case of severe mud fever the hair has been trimmed to allow for treatment

keeping the area as clean and dry as practicable. If the pony is stabled at night he can have clean gamgee and dry bandages put on his legs, to warm and dry them. The gamgee should be thrown away each day to stop perpetuating the infection. For rain scald, you should put on a clean summer sheet every day underneath his top rug and this should be washed daily in very hot water.

Veterinary treatment is not usually necessary unless hair loss is severe or if swelling occurs at the site or the horse has a raised temperature. Tea tree cream is a very useful herbal remedy and the area can also be cleaned with a pint of warm water containing five or six drops of neat tea tree oil.

MELANOMA

Melanoma is usually only seen in old grey horses. It is a form of skin cancer and usually first appears as raised black lumps about the size of a pea. The lumps may increase and grow together to form much bigger tumours or they may just stay there exactly as they were when you first saw them. Never ever touch a melanoma or try to bathe it or do anything else. If it should get damaged or rubbed by tack or rugs just treat it as a wound and keep it clean and apply wound powder until it dries up again. If you are worried or lumps appear to start to spread rapidly you must consult your vet. It is usually definitely not an immediate death sentence for any pony even if it is cancer. Many ponies live perfectly happily with a number of melanomas on their body.

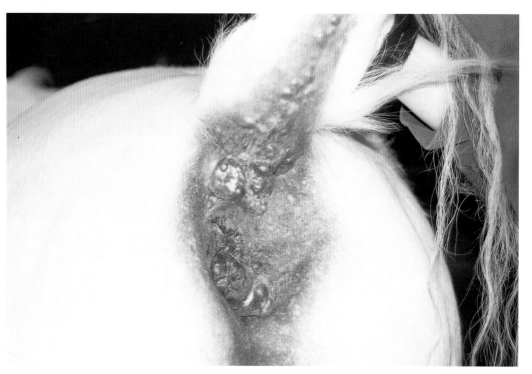

Melanoma

RINGWORM

Ringworm is a highly contagious fungal disease which can also easily spread to humans. It appears as a circular bald patch, often on the face. Get diagnosis from your vet and then

94

isolate the animal. Everything that comes in contact with him must be disinfected including his tack and his grooming kit must be kept separate. You must disinfect your hands thoroughly after touching him or wear disposable gloves. Tea tree cream makes a good emergency treatment but veterinary anti-fungal lotions and creams will effect a much quicker recovery.

SWEET ITCH

This shows as an irritation in the mane and or tail and in very bad cases on the sides of the neck and the face as well. It is caused by biting from the Culicoides midge to which some animals are hypersensitive. Prevention is always best. Affected animals should be stabled at dusk in warm weather and all day in humid, dull but warm weather. Fly repellent should be used at all times and renewed regularly. The stable should be kept clear of cobwebs and several sticky fly strips hung up especially near the doors and windows. The door and window should be covered with a net curtain. Local treatment is with cooling lotion such as calamine or the rubbing on of fresh mint leaves. In serious cases the vet will need to be called to administer steroids.

Sweet itch

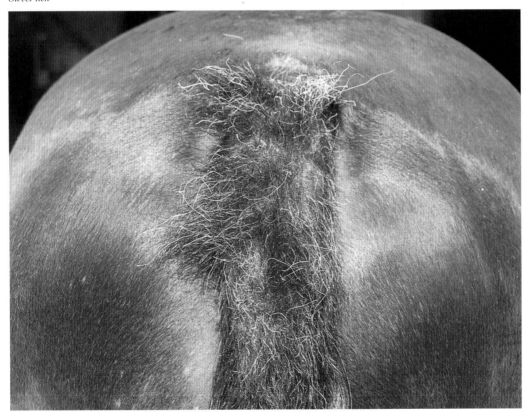

Rugs and other garments

THE NEW ZEALAND RUG

Most native ponies have their own built in New Zealand rug – better known as their coat. However, New Zealand rugs are invaluable for the pony which is clipped and working in the winter. They come in various fabrics nowadays but the basic idea is a tough waterproof rug to be worn outdoors. If you have a very active pony look out for cross surcingles which appear on most rugs now. If using a rug on a daily basis, you should really have a spare one. It is sometimes impossible to dry the rug overnight and if you put it on again in the morning wet and by now also cold then it will be stiff and uncomfortable and the pony may well attempt to get it off.

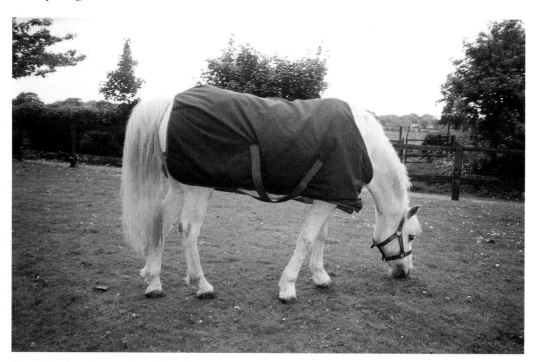

New Zealand rug for wet and/or cold weather and also for a pony which has been clipped

Leg straps, if they are fitted need to be kept soft and clean to avoid them rubbing the sensitive inside of the legs. Leather straps should be well soaked in neatsfoot oil regularly, so that they can be washed off on a daily basis in wet weather. Nylon straps should be washed and given a soak in fabric conditioner. This will keep them soft and help them to stay clean longer – hopefully!

All straps and buckles and other fittings should be checked regularly and repaired or replaced as necessary. The rug should fit properly. It should be snug round the shoulders to avoid rubbing as much as possible. There should be no gaping at the front. Loose fitting at the front may mean that the rug could get caught on the fence or that if the pony lies down he might get his knee into the front of the rug and be unable to get up.

STABLE RUGS

These come in every material, colour and design imaginable. Washable fabric is always the easiest to cope with but may be less durable. Jute is almost completely out of fashion but can last for years and be very cheap initially. Cross surcingles are again the best fastening. Some rugs come with a separate panel at the front, meaning that there are two front fastenings, one on each side. This can be very useful for native ponies with a very wide chest.

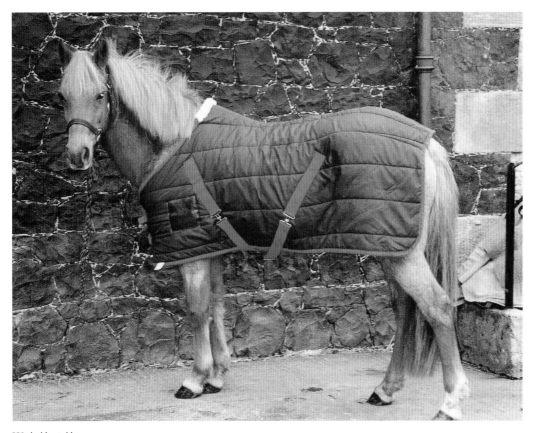

Washable stable rug

SUMMER SHEETS

Summer sheets are a useful addition to your pony's wardrobe. Made of heavy duty cotton material and most useful if fitted with their own cross surcingles, this rug can be used all the year round. In summer it is useful for travelling and for keeping the pony clean after bathing. In winter it can be used under other rugs for keeping the top rugs clean. Being thinner it is much more easily washed and dried and can therefore save work.

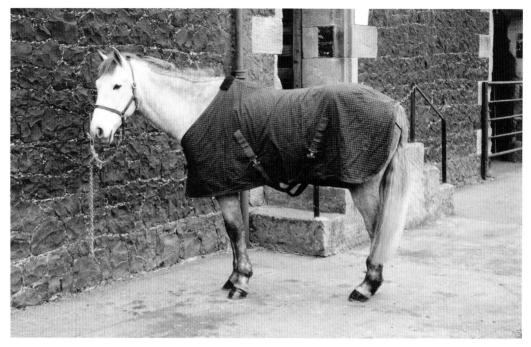

Summer sheet with crossed surcingles

Partly clipped pony with sweat rug

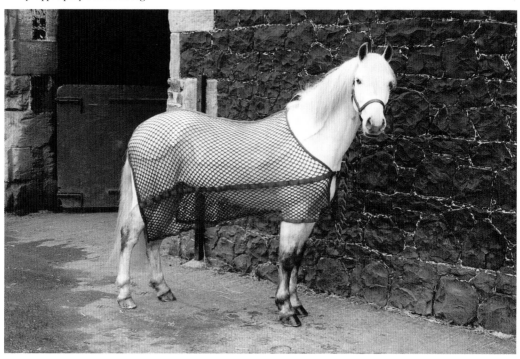

SWEAT RUGS AND COOLERS

All ridden ponies need a rug of this type. Native ponies working with their full coat or even when they are partly clipped can get very sweaty. If you intend to turn them out after work it is essential to dry off the coat to avoid chilling. There are some very advanced fabrics now being used for cooler rugs which facilitate quick drying. Although somewhat expensive they can be invaluable.

HOODS

Stretch hoods are becoming increasingly popular amongst native pony exhibitors. They can keep the mane lying flat and stop a pony rubbing if he has a tendency to itch. However, for a pony with sweet itch they can be too warming and make matters much worse.

BIBS AND UNDER RUGS

These are made of silk or other slippery material and are designed to stop rugs rubbing.

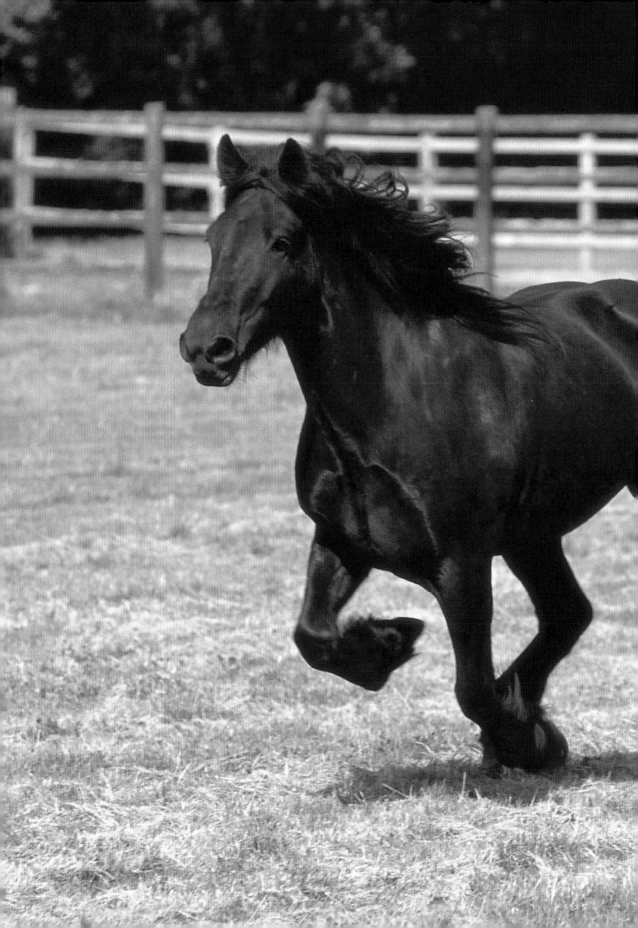

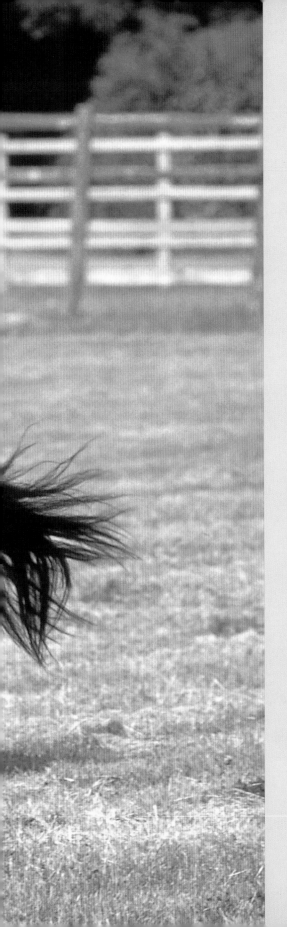

6

Breeding

The very first question you should ask yourself as you look at your mare and imagine her with a foal is 'Am I prepared for the responsibility?' The responsibility of bringing another equine into the world when hundreds go for meat every week. The responsibility of keeping the mare and foal for at least eighteen months, during pregnancy and whilst the foal is at foot. The responsibility of the inevitable veterinary bills. The responsibility of finding the foal a job to do and possibly a good home if you decide not to keep him yourself. All these factors should be considered even before you look for a potential sire.

You will also need a stable. Of course, native ponies can foal outside and are indeed often better to do so if the weather is reasonable, but it can snow in April; the mare and/or the foal might be ill making a stable an essential. You will also need good pasture with good fencing – a safe place for your baby to play! If you have other horses you will also need somewhere that your mare can be alone with her foal. Many mares do not bother about others – after all they were designed to foal within their herd but some, especially first time mothers, need to sort themselves out without having to worry about anything else.

You will need to be prepared to sit up with your mare when she is about to foal, especially if it is her first foal. This is almost impossible if she is not in a field or stable near to your home.

You have to be sure that your mare is good enough to warrant all this effort and expense. If you are not sure and she is not proven in the show ring then do ask the independent advice of someone who knows what they are talking about. Breeding from a mare with conformational faults does your chosen breed no good at all. Be careful too of breeding from a mare with 'psychological' problems. An extremely timid mare will probably pass this on to her foal. A bad tempered mare will no doubt give the foal a hard time. Some experts say that a predisposition to vices such as crib biting, windsucking and box walking are hereditary. Whilst there is no scientific evidence to prove this there is certainly some anecdotal evidence around. Indeed, the author has two ponies by the same stallion who both windsuck. In more than forty years I have never had any others with this vice. However, I know three other ponies also by the same stallion and these all have the vice too. It is certainly not conclusive evidence but surely enough to make you think twice if your mare does have a stable vice.

Fashions versus traditions in breeding

The breed standards as they are today have evolved over the last one hundred years. Height limits now seem to have settled into an agreed format. Only very minor changes have taken place in standards over say the last fifty years. However, fashions within these standards seem to change all the time. Take for example the Welsh Mountain Pony. If you look back at famous stallions such as Greylight (foaled in 1900) his head today would be considered very plain. Mares of that time too had much larger, plainer heads and were also well up to the height limit of 12hh. Their acton was powerful, with strong shoulder movement and some lifting of the knee. The very worst examples of ponies with faults bred in have ridiculously small heads with ears the size of mouse ears. It is almost impossible to keep a bridle on them. They skim along the floor like ballet dancers, pointing their toes in a very pretty manner. To get up a mountainside would be an impossibility. Yet these ponies became like this because breeders were trying to get the 'small' head and 'bold' eye of the breed standard together with an action 'well away in front'.

This is a good example of breeding going too far in trying to produce show champions. Mating mother with son or daughter with father to bring out desirable characteristics is a good way of also producing freaks, where a desirable characteristic – say a small head – then produces such a small head that there is no room for a brain. It can also produce other undesirable characteristics such as mental problems and inherent weakness.

Having said all this a good stallion with good conformation will always be a good one, even as fashions come and go.

Choosing your sire

Much can be done to improve the chances of breeding a champion with careful choice of a sire. If your mare has slight faults – and do be honest about them – then a sire can be chosen who could counter this. For example, if she has a plain head, a pretty head on the stallion may well produce an acceptable combination of the two in the foal. If you are a novice breeder, do take the advice of an expert, preferably one without a stallion they can persuade you to use. Certain bloodlines combine well with others and only vast experience will give you this knowledge. Certain stallions are 'in fashion' at any one time and stock got by them will have a slightly higher value. You should also work out whether you want your mare to run out with her husband or to be covered in hand. Some stallions do both, but some only do one or the other and your choice may be affected by this. If she is covered in hand she may well stay a shorter time at the stud which will affect costs. Every stud owner has slightly different ideas about what they want from owners of visiting mares and this should be discussed when you go to visit your chosen stallion(s).

If you are thinking of covering your native mare in any given year and you do not have a stallion in mind then do visit the early stallion shows which are held in various venues all over the country. You can see the best stallions 'on parade' in the show ring and may get a chance to speak to their owners. You will, however, have to act swiftly after this to get your mare covered in time.

Many stallion owners require visiting mares to be screened for Equine Contagious Metritis and will not accept a mare without a certificate. In the Horserace Betting Levy Board Code of Practice which was formulated in 1977 specific measures are laid down to prevent the spread of this disease in Thoroughbred and native stock. Your breed society will have a copy of the code and will be able to give you specific advice.

The season

The season, or oestrus as it is more properly called, occurs from when the pony is approximately two years until very old age. The oestrus occurs from about March to July every fourteen to twenty-eight days and lasts for two to eight days. Mares vary considerably in their reaction to being 'in season'. In some it passes virtually unnoticed and in other they will become screaming mad things yelling at any gelding even seen on the distant horizon and generally being unmanageable. Thankfully the majority fall on middle ground with young mares being slightly more irritable and possibly putting their tails up and passing small amounts of urine, especially when you brush their back end.

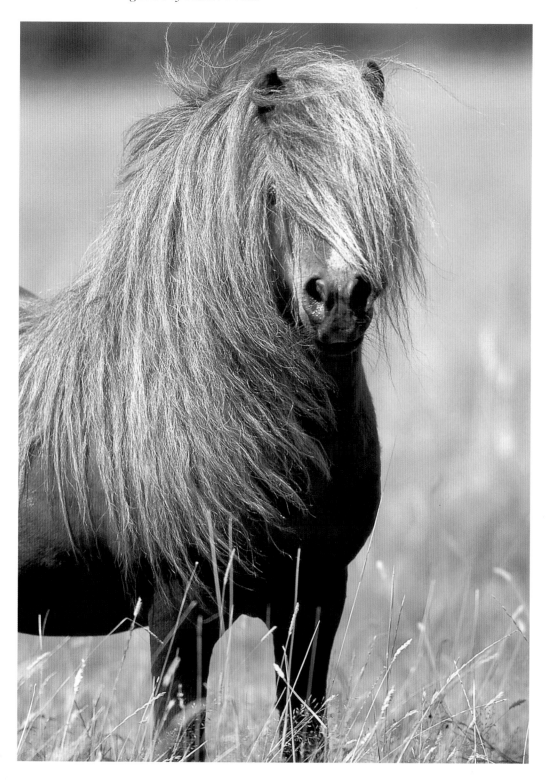

If you wish to mate your mare you should make a point of watching her seasons and knowing when she is ready. Service takes place around the ninth day, but by this time she should be safely ensconced at the stallion's premises and the stud owner will know exactly what to do. Every stud wants you to bring your mare at a slightly different time. If she is to run out with the stallion timing is not quite so crucial. Many native mares will come in season anyway when turned out with the stallion. The mere sight of him gets them in the mood! 'Walking in' with mare means just that – you take your mares to the stallion's premises when you think she is ready and she gets covered and taken home again. This really only works for the experienced owner who knows her mare well.

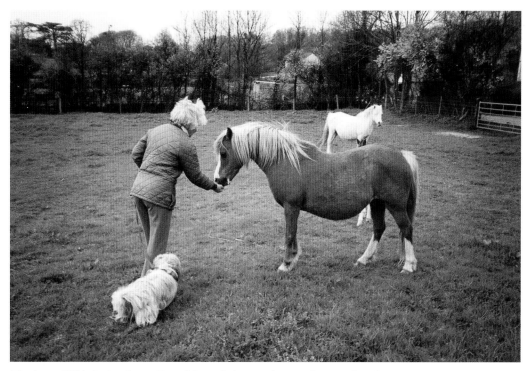

The famous Welsh Section A mare Bengad Rose of Sharon at home at the Bengad Stud

Care of the mare during pregnancy and foaling

The most important decision to make as this momentous occasion approaches is where the event is going to take place. If the weather is fine and your native mare is fit and well then an outside foaling should produce no problems at all. Indeed the mare can walk about whilst labour is in progress and can get up and down as the birth approaches without any fear of

Shetland stallion at Stepley Stud

hurting herself. If the weather is cold or wet then she may have to be confined indoors. A large stable, well bedded down with clean straw looks very nice to us. However, some native mares will not have this at any price and you will just have to be guided by your instincts. Native mares have been known to hold on to their foal until they get put out rather than foal indoors. They have also been known to jump fences to get away from their companions and give birth in peace. Watch your mare carefully so that you can make appropriate decisions as and when necessary.

Pregnancy lasts for an average of 340 days. The pregnant mare needs to be kept in good condition but not allowed to become too gross which may affect foaling. Worming in an important factor to consider. It should be done every six to eight weeks during the pregnancy and the worming product used should be suitable for pregnant mares. She can be ridden lightly until the last three months but should not be galloped or jumped or ridden so long that she gets stressed.

During the first eight months or so of pregnancy the growing foetus makes very little demand on the mare. However, she should be kept in good health and fed in order to keep her this way. If grazing is limited she must have supplementary feed, together with a good vitamin and mineral supplement, if a proprietary mix is not fed. During the last three months of the pregnancy the foal is growing much more quickly and feeding should therefore increase accordingly. If the spring grass is good a native mare may well keep in good condition without any extra food but in a cold wet spring or if your grazing is poor you should look to giving her extra food so that she is in peak condition when the foal is due. If you wish to show her with the foal at foot it is especially important that she does not lose too much ground by the foaling.

As foaling gets near the mare's udder will increase in size. A secretion known as 'waxing' will usually occur during the last few days. However, it should be borne in mind that some mares foal without showing either of these signs. In the last couple of days the muscles around the tail will relax, appearing slack from behind. When foaling is imminent the mare will become restless, possibly swishing her tail and getting up and lying down. This is the time to make sure that she is in a safe place for the foaling and not near to any hazards if she is outside. Stay with her at this time. If she shows signs of straining for more than half an hour or is getting distressed or sweating without anything happening then call the vet. You should have put him or her on notice that you have a pregnant mare and that the foal is expected on such and such a date. Have hot water and a towel ready (and as good a light source as possible if it is night). In a normal foaling the front end comes first – the forelegs with the head lying along them. The membrane may cover its face and if this is the case puncture it by hand – it usually splits easily – and remove it from the foal's eyes and nose. A foal can smother very quickly if this is not done, even if half of the foal is not yet delivered. If you are watching your mare and the hind legs come out first or the head without the front feet then the vet should be called immediately. The foal may still be born safely, especially if it is small but do not take any risks. Never attempt to pull the foal out if you are inexperienced. You may do more harm than good.

When the foal is finally delivered the mare will probably lie down for some time and appear exhausted. This is normal but if she is not up within fifteen minutes there is cause for concern. The foal usually gets up fairly quickly and some foals are already looking for the udder within a couple of minutes. The umbilical cord will sever as he gets up or as he moves. The afterbirth should be delivered within an hour or two after the birth. You will need to spread it out and check that it appears whole. If you have any doubts save it for the vet to look at. If the afterbirth has not appeared after three hours you will need veterinary help.

After foaling the mare will need to produce several gallons of milk a day for her foal. Her needs can be equated to a pony in regular work at least. She will also need increased amounts of calcium and phosphorus. These can be given by feeding a complete mix designed for broodmares or by offering feed with an added measure of bonemeal. It is important not to change the mare's diet suddenly during lactation as the change may affect the foal. Occasionally a mare will reject her foal. This is most likely with a first-time mother, but even in this situation is unusual. It may be possible to hold the mare on a headcollar and let the foal suck whilst she gets used to the idea. If you still have problems, then do seek veterinary help urgently. A foal goes downhill very quickly if he does not feed very soon. He needs the

first milk (colostrum) to help set him up for life. The foal's navel should be treated with an appropriate antiseptic spray and then checked regularly for signs of infection.

If you lose a foal or lose the mare during foaling then do get in touch immediately with the National Foaling Bank (see page 140 for address) who may well find you an orphan foal who needs a mother or a mare who has successfully reared other foals but who has lost this one. It is possible to hand-rear a foal and there are special milk formulas available for this purpose, but there are so many other things that a foal learns from a mare that it is always best to keep hand rearing as a last resort.

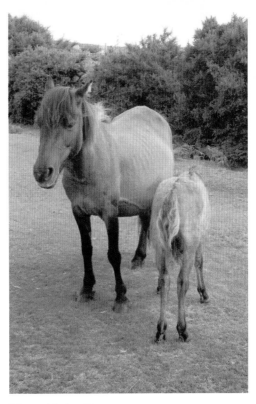

Mare and foal on Dartmoor

If you are unlucky enough to get a deformed foal or one which is very weak or sickly then you should seek veterinary advice. A deformed foal is never going to have a useful life.

The foal should pass its first dropping within an hour of birth and they can be a startling orange or very black in colour – this is normal. The foal may have a certain amount of scouring when the mare comes into season at around a week after the birth. By 'scouring' we mean an extreme looseness of the bowels which is very dangerous to young foals because of the great risk of dehydration. If this is severe or prolonged you will need veterinary help.

The foal can go out into the field in fine weather with his dam from the first day. Unless he has been born outside and has adequate shelter, you should keep him indoors in very bad weather. He can be weaned from around six months onwards, but for show stock he can be left with his mother throughout his first winter (as long as she is not pregnant again). This will give him the very best start in life. Most foals start eating grass very quickly and can be given hard food by way of a special youngstock mix, when their mother is fed, from about six weeks onwards.

Weaning

Weaning takes place at any time from six months onwards. The foal will be spending time away from his mother if she is being ridden again. Incidentally riding the mare does help to dry her milk up. It is always easier to separate the mare and foal finally if the foal has a companion to go with. This can be another foal or it can be an older quiet mare who will 'look after' him and teach him some manners. The mare will shout for the foal for the first few days or she may not seem to be bothered at all – every mare is different. It does help if the foal is out of earshot. If they can hear each other call it will perpetuate the bond. It is best to leave a mare and foal apart for several weeks at least, even if you need to put them back together eventually. For native ponies, if the mare is not in foal again, it can often give the foal a very good start in life if he is left with his mother for the first winter. It will do the mare no harm and will give her an opportunity to teach her foal much more about life.

Care of foals and young stock

THE YEARLING

The foal becomes a yearling on the first of January following his birth. By now he will have usually been weaned from his mother and will be growing well. The watchwords at this age are education and feeding. His education should be continuing. He should lead easily; have his feet trimmed without too much fuss and generally be easy to handle. Every young pony is lively and can be difficult sometimes but a general trend towards good behaviour is what you are working towards.

His diet will consist of grass and/or hay depending on the season of the year and the weather. Concentrates are not absolutely essential, but for the best growth and for show stock, they are useful. The very best way to feed concentrates at this age is from a ready prepared mix designed especially for youngstock, unless you are able to calculate accurately what nutrients are required by individuals.

Having spent most of his first year with his mother the yearling is now ready to learn about being a grown-up pony. He should by now lead easily, going away from the others on his own. He will have met the blacksmith to have his feet trimmed. He will be eating some hard food and should be given a ration especially designed for foals or a supplement for young horses.

If you intend to show him and have not ventured out to foal shows, remember that the earlier you start the easier it will be. Anyone who has shown a three-year-old Welsh cob colt will tell you this! He will need to get used to travelling and to the strange sights and sounds of the show ring. He will also need to see some of the outside world. Keeping youngstock in a field next to a road helps to get them used to traffic without putting them at any risk.

Regular grooming and handling does much to establish a good relationship between your young pony and human beings.

If a ridden career is his destiny then putting a rug on him now and again will be useful even if he is not rugged up. It helps him to be used to something on his back. Bathing is another occurrence that he should get used to, but do make sure it is a warm sunny summer day. Youngsters catch cold much more quickly than older ponies.

He will need to continue to be wormed four times a year and to be vaccinated annually. If your horses never leave the premises then tetanus vaccination is adequate but protection against flu viruses should be added if you are going showing or anywhere else.

TWO-AND THREE-YEAR OLDS

Your pony's education should continue whilst he grows up. By the time he is three years old he should be leading quietly both at home and out on the roads. He should wear a saddle and bridle and larger breeds can begin to be ridden away. He should travel; wear a rug; stand still for the blacksmith and generally be a settled, confident and (mostly!) well behaved individual.

Selling

Having bred your foal and possibly kept him until he is two or three years old you will have put in a great deal of time and effort – not to say emotional commitment. So how do you find him a new home? The best solution is obviously to sell him to someone whom you already know. If this is not possible there are several other options.

You could advertise him in *Horse & Hound*. This is by far the best known magazine in the horse world. Every week it carries adverts for horses and ponies for sale and it is to this publication that most people turn when they are in the market for a pony. Word your advertisement carefully but absolutely truthfully. For example you can say something like 'prizewinner in the show ring'. You do not need to mention that it was at the local small show. However, if you say prizewinner at county level this must mean that he has been in the first four or five in his class at a county show. If he has vices than you must declare them to a potential purchaser, whether they ask or not. You do not however need to mention them in the advert! They may fall in love with him and be prepared to disregard the vice.

Unfortunately, prospective purchasers will telephone at all times of the day (and sometimes) night and will make arrangements to view and not turn up. You must be prepared to be philosophical about this. When they do come to view you should have the pony confined in a stable or at least tied up somewhere, unless they have specifically asked to see him in the field. He should be clean and tidy but most potential customers do not necessarily need him to be turned out as for a show. In fact, this almost looks suspect – you may have something to hide and be trying to dazzle the customer with gloss and glitter. If he is a ridden pony your tack should be clean and well fitting. It should be remembered that the fit of a bridle or headcollar can do much to enhance the head of a pony.

For an unbroken pony there should be somewhere to trot him up easily. If he moves best on a hard surface then this is the place to do it. For ridden ponies there should be a menage or paddock that is not several feet deep in mud. If he is not safe on the road, then do say so, or at least before a potential purchaser takes him on the road. Anyone who compromises the safety of a potential purchaser in an effort to sell the pony risks being sued if anything goes wrong.

There are several vices which you are required to declare if selling a pony through a saleyard and should be declared in any case to safeguard yourself if you are selling privately. These vices are rearing, windsucking, crib-biting and weaving. Other vices which you should declare if you are selling privately are bolting; dung-eating; rug tearing and such problems as being difficult to catch, load or shoe. If your pony has any other glaring problems such as being terrified of sheep or the clippers or whatever then you would do well to declare this and should certainly be truthful if asked.

SELLING THROUGH THE SALE YARD

The breed societies all have sales for registered ponies at various times of the year. The National Pony Society also holds sales of registered ponies and registered part breds. Various auctioneers hold regular sales all over the country with widely varying standards. You should enquire from your breed society which of these sales are of a good standard, before you enter your pony. Sales are advertised in *Horse & Hound* and other equestrian publications. Smaller sales will be advertised in your local paper. There are sales up and down the country which anyone who cares the tiniest bit for their pony should avoid like the plague. The ponies go to other dealers who trail them round other sales or sell them on for meat. If you have any doubts about a sale yard you should contact your local RSPCA. They provide a welfare officer at all sales and will give you the necessary advice.

Having chosen your sale and ensured

that it is of a high standard, the next move is to get your pony entered. This has to be done well in advance if a catalogue is to be produced. There will be a fee to pay. Some potential buyers may want to see your pony at home before the sale and if the auctioneers permit this you can put your telephone number in the catalogue.

On the day of the sale arrive well before the sale starts. You will know what lot number you are so can judge the time you will be needed in the ring. The staff at most sale yards are well geared up to help the first time seller, so confess your ignorance and they will keep an eye on you and make sure all goes well. You can put a reserve price on your pony. This is a price below which you would not sell him. Watch the auctioneer,

because if bidding goes very close to your reserve he may look at you to see if you will accept it. If you put no reserve on your pony could in theory sell for less than it cost you to enter him in the sale. His new owners will usually come over and introduce themselves after the sale. You will need to give them a headcollar and rope to take him away. His papers will have been lodged with the auctioneer well before the sale.

Selling in a sale yard works well for studs who have a number of ponies for sale and no time to show prospective buyers round one at a time. It should not be used as a dumping ground for ponies with problems. You will only condemn them, unless you are very lucky, to turning up again and again in other sales.

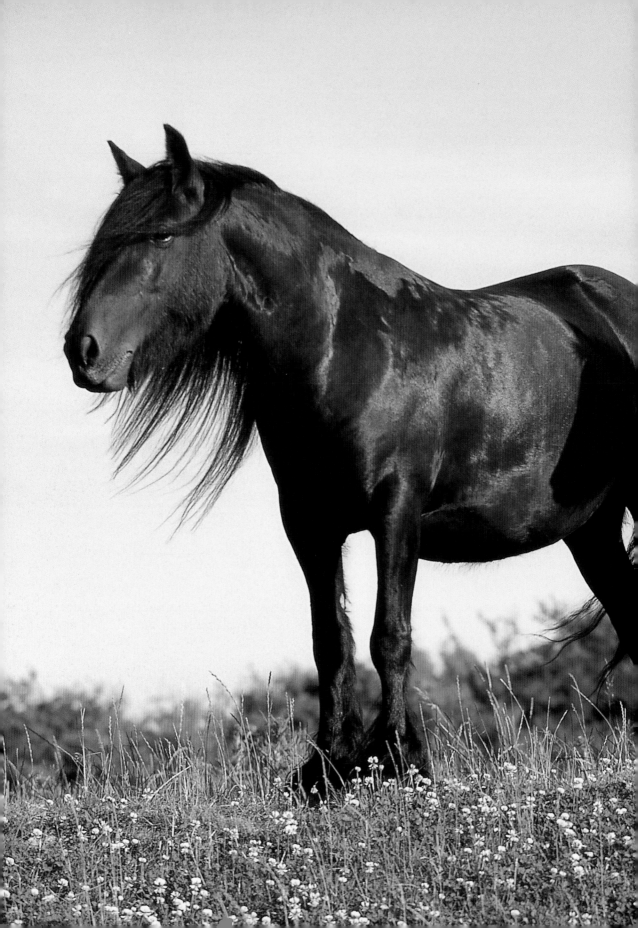

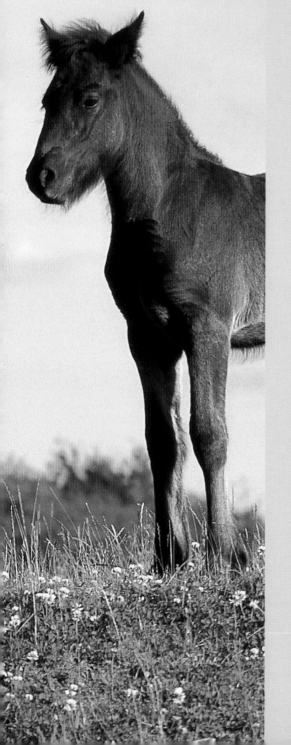

7

Preparing to Show

Showing is lots of fun – and lots of disappointment. It is also very, very hard work. You cannot expect to make any profit from showing your pony in a direct way. Even if he wins a big championship, the prize money often barely covers the entry fee and travelling expenses. However, if you intend to breed from your pony or you want to sell him on, with 'miles on his clock' then you can add to his value by winning prizes especially if these are at county level shows. If you sell a pony having qualified him for one or more of the big championships then you will certainly add to his desirability and often to his value as well.

Shows, championships and entries

Shows are advertised in publications such as *Horse & Hound* on a regular basis. This publication in particular has a two part 'show number' in the early spring, which has very comprehensive listings of shows of

Fell mare and foal

all sizes. You should send for schedules of all the shows which may interest you within acceptable travelling distance. Some of the bigger shows have closing dates for entries two or three months ahead and they are usually very strict about not accepting entries after that date. The major championships for native ponies are held under the rules of the National Pony Society and Ponies UK. If you are serious about showing you would need to join both of these organisations (see address list for details) at the beginning of the year. Currently, for some of the National Pony Society championships you will also need to register the pony and obtain a competition record card for him. All societies change their rules sometimes so it is imperative that you obtain a rule book and check the current requirements very carefully.

Judges at these championship qualifying shows will be on the society panel of judges and *should* be capable of judging all other breeds besides the one or two that they specialise in. This is not always the case and judges can also be accused of favouring their own breed in a mixed class. However, this is not by all means the case and indeed the author's own Welsh Section C took the Picton Supreme championship over a Highland Pony in front of a Highland judge. If you are going to be consistently unhappy with the way judging is done then you should give up showing altogether. There is very often no rhyme or reason to the results no matter what level you compete at.

If you do not intend to compete at this exalted level then almost every show now

has 'Mountain and Moorland' classes either ridden or in-hand or both. If the show is not under the rules of any society then the judge may well not be the greatest expert on the breed standard requirements of different breeds but hopefully they will have an eye for conformation and conformation is the same whether your animal is a Shetland Pony or a hunter.

Some shows take entries on the day, sometimes with a percentage added to the entry fee for late entries. If you intend to do this you must arrive at the show in time to queue to hand in your entry. It is no good standing in the line at the secretary's office when your class starts!

Starting with youngstock

If you have an older pony that has been shown before you can skip this next section. If you have a youngster that you intend to show either in-hand or later on under saddle then there are some important points to remember. The atmosphere at a showground is absolutely electrifying to all but the most laid-back horses when they first encounter it. There are other horses galloping around and jumping and every instinct tells them to run with the herd. Add to these unexpected noises such as loudspeakers coupled with large lorries driving very close to them in the lorry park and you can see how any youngster would at least be excited. Native ponies tend in general to be sensible and your pony will soon get used to showgrounds if you make the effort to take him to as many events as necessary before you actually take him in

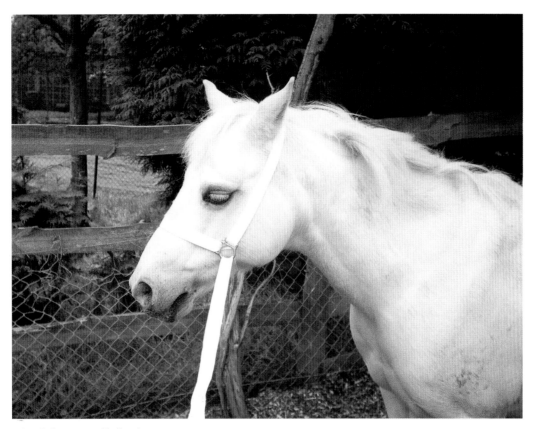

White halter not suitable for colts over two years

the ring. You should make sure that you have him under proper control. This means using a bridle if you will need it not a flimsy halter. Lead him around the showground until he settles, then if you have no other ponies to show you should load him up and take him home again. Take him to another event again as soon as possible. It does not matter if it is showjumping or something which he may not ever do, as long as it is an 'event'. The atmosphere will be similar.

Schooling at home is vital if you are not to make a complete fool of yourself when you first appear in the ring. This applies also to in-hand exhibitors. The in-hand pony should learn to stand on command and to lead quietly but willingly when asked to do so.

A colt must get used to wearing a bit very quickly. Two-year-old colts and over must be shown in a bridle under most rules. He can start with a little nylon straight bar or jointed bit with brass rings to match an in-hand bridle. By three he should have progressed to a stallion bit, especially if he is one of the larger breeds. Some people like to show in what is called 'stallion tack'. This consists of a bridle, side reins and a roller, with or without a crupper. If you intend to use the items in the ring, you will have to practise at home. The crupper particularly offends some males!

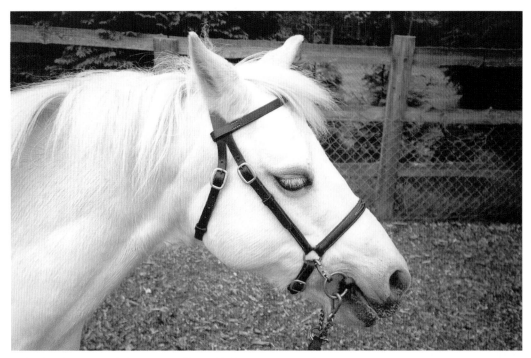

In-hand bridle with straight bar nylon snaffle suitable for mare or young colt

In-hand bridle without bit for mare or filly

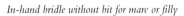

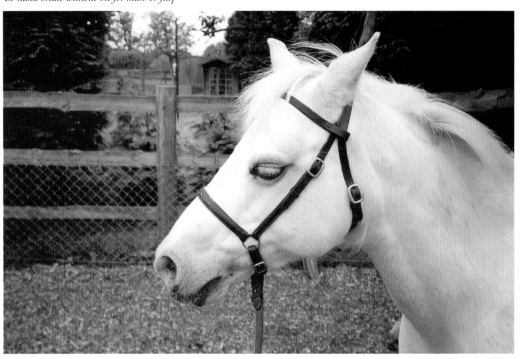

Early Training

If you are breaking in your own pony, everything should be done from the beginning with his eventual future in mind. Great care should be taken so that he never goes 'sour' from doing too much of one thing, especially endless schooling in circles in a menage or the same corner of a field. Nothing spoils a pony more than if he goes round the ring with a thoroughly grumpy expression on his face and his legs going as if they were full of lead. He needs to come into the ring 'smiling' with his ears pricked and his expression alert. He should move freely, with a 'spring in his step' and just look as if he is really enjoying himself. All breeds of native ponies can have such enormous presence and everything should be done to encourage this. Just stand and watch a class of native ponies and you will see what I mean when I say that the right attitude on the part of the pony goes a long way to getting him noticed by the judge.

When you are first training him, it will be very useful to show him in-hand, even if you only do it a few times. It will get him used to the showground and to behaving himself in company. Teach him to stand square right from the beginning. Praise him when he does right and walk him forward a pace or two to adjust his feet when he is not square. Lead him on the left-hand side and ask him to walk with his shoulder level with you. If he drags behind encourage him with a long stick held in your left hand and used behind your back to reach his flank. If he pulls, talk to him in your most soothing voice. If he is

consistently difficult to handle, then he could need less food and more time in the field. If you are inexperienced in handling young horses then do seek professional help, before faults which may be difficult to eradicate later get established.

The paces and action of a pony can do much to attract the judge's eye and the pace most used in the ring is actually the walk. Whether in-hand or ridden he may well walk round for some considerable time whilst the judge forms first impressions and he will be walking again when final decisions are made. He should therefore be taught from the beginning to walk out freely and strongly. Lazy walkers should be long-reined so that their pace can be driven from behind and encouraged to lengthen whilst speed can be restricted by the reins.

Correctly fitted snaffle bridle

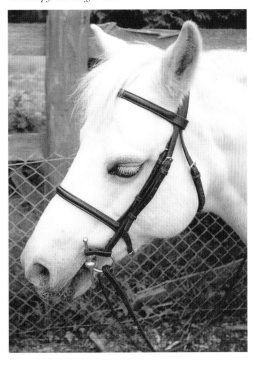

A pony that walks with tiny quick steps needs a hill! He will have to lengthen his stride to walk up and down hill and with time this will become easier and more natural for him to do on the flat. It is an important fact to remember that the front action can be greatly improved by work on the back end. Quite often ponies go in the ring with their head held too high, their back hollowed out and their hocks almost tripping up the pony behind. By always encouraging your pony to use himself you will avoid these problems.

Even a young pony can be led over a pole on the ground. This will help later when he comes to jump and by gradually increasing the number of poles to a small grid you can encourage use of all legs and the back in negotiating the obstacles. He also cannot step over the poles with any accuracy if his head is too high to see where he is going. He will naturally lower his head to look at the poles, thus giving him a better shape altogether.

All equines of any age must not be allowed to get bored. The work pattern should vary from day to day to keep them interested. A walk down to the post-box to post letters; being tied up in the yard whilst others are shod; being taken to a show even if he is not to be shown and so on and so on. All these activities are part of his education and development. Every aspect of your pony's training should be carried out with a view to the future. By the same token, just as horses learn quickly what you want of them so they also learn quickly bad habits and frightening experiences can be difficult to overcome. Every ridden pony should be completely safe in traffic. You

might think that you will never have to take him on the road, but if you show him for example, you will meet lorries in the lorry park. If you are riding across farm land you will undoubtedly meet tractors and possibly even four wheel drive vehicles. If you want to sell him in the future and he is not used to traffic he could prove difficult to sell. The best way to accustom your young pony to traffic is to start by putting him in a paddock by a busy road, especially if he is with older ponies who will ignore the road in preference for the grass. If this is not possible take him out in-hand, wearing a bridle for control and with an older pony for company. Lead him along confidently and if he shies at traffic just keep going, talking to him and reassuring him with your voice. Never punish a pony for demonstrating fear, it will just make him more fearful.

By the age of three the larger natives should be ready to be lightly backed. Smaller ponies are better left until four. Start by putting a roller and bridle on him, if he has not come across these items before (he may have had a roller with a rug and he may have been shown in a bridle). Use an old bridle with no noseband and a jointed snaffle with a good thick mouthpiece. You can get special breaking bits, with rollers to encourage mouthing but most ponies take well to an ordinary bit. Leave it on just for a few minutes to begin with, gradually building up time. The roller can be substituted for an old saddle and the girth gradually tightened until he wears it without objection in the stable. He can then be led about wearing this tack.

It is vital never to rush your pony. If

things go wrong then go back at least one stage to something he is comfortable with. Your patience at this stage will be rewarded many times over in the future. If you are a person of excitable disposition or lacking in patience then do not even bother to try and break your pony yourself – send him to a professional.

Gradually introduce the stirrups to the saddle, leaving them hanging down to touch his side as he walks. When he is going happily in his tack both at walk and trot and possibly being lunged or long-reined in it, it is time to mount. The pony should be held by a competent person and the potential rider should have a mounting block. The rider should lean across the pony patting him and talking to him. For a few minutes at a time, more and more weight can be put on the back until the full weight of the rider is across the pony. He can then be led forward a step or two with the rider still sideways so that he can easily dismount if there is an adverse reaction from the pony. After this has been accomplished on a number of occasions, the rider can swing a leg across and sit astride. The pony can then be led about like this. As you can see the breaking of a pony is usually easily accomplished if each step is taken carefully and patiently.

At no time at this stage should the rider touch the pony's mouth at all. Only when he is going forward confidently for some time can he be expected to accept the bit and contact from the rider. Far too many ponies end up unhappy in their mouth because they were hauled around by the reins before they really knew what was expected of them.

The in-hand class

The format of the in-hand class is as follows. Competitors enter the ring at walk, leading their exhibit on its nearside. They will walk round the outside of the ring, in a clockwise direction. After several circuits the steward will station himself or herself at one corner of the ring. The next competitor to get to her will stop and all the others will line up behind. Do not get too close! Each in turn will trot their pony on, going along the side of the ring, past the judge and slowing to a walk well in time before they get to the waiting ponies. When all have done this, the steward will walk the whole class on again. Watch the steward who will call the ponies into line usually in a provisional order. Occasionally the whole class will be called into line together. Each pony will then come out individually and stand before the judge. As for ridden classes, competitors should not chat to the judge or boast of the pony's previous achievements. A polite greeting and answering of questions is all that is required. The judge will then send you away to do an individual show. This is done exactly as for the in-hand part of a ridden show, unless the judge asks you to do something else and this does happen occasionally. Sometimes in a big class the judge will have two ponies out at once to look at. Whatever format the class takes, just keep alert and watch the steward and you should not make any mistakes.

After all the ponies have been seen, the steward will walk them on round again and a final decision will be made. The prizewinners leave the ring on the right rein at a trot. The others walk out directly to the exit.

What happens in a ridden class?

All of the ponies will enter the ring at walk. They should spread out to take up the whole of the outside track of the ring. Children especially tend to go in a follow-the-leader riding school style, so that all the ponies are in only part of the ring and all bunched up so closely that they cannot be properly seen. It is quite in order to either circle into a space or to wait at a corner to give the pony in front more room. What is not acceptable and is sadly getting very common is to trot across the centre of the ring in extended trot, passing so close to the judge that you almost run them over, thus hoping to attract early attention. It will only annoy most judges.

Your walk should be free and brisk without hurrying. Your pony should be on the bit carrying it lightly in his mouth and with his head in the correct position. He should be alert and 'smiling'. Watch the steward. At some point he or she will tell you to trot on. Do this immediately and get your pony settled into a rhythm before he comes round in front of the judge the next time. As you go in front of the judge ensure that he is doing his very best trot. This may well include an element of extension. You can relax as you go behind the judge but do remember that she may turn round and look behind her at any time, so you cannot slop along. The steward will then ask the class to canter. If you cannot be sure of your pony going on the correct leg then wait

until you get to a corner. The canter can often seem like a cavalry charge, especially in a large breeds class in a small ring. Some ponies can be very panicky in these circumstances and buck or bolt and many a class has to be stopped whilst a pony is recovered or a rider rescued. You should have practised having your pony in a noisy fast-moving crowd at home or should at least stand him by the ring a few times to watch before you get him in the fray.

Most judges ask the class to come back to trot, go across the centre and then canter on the other rein. The trot across the centre will give you a good opportunity to show an extension. Some judges want a class to gallop. This particularly applies to larger breeds. You should be prepared for this. The class will then be brought back to walk. Do not slop along! Come into walk with your pony under control and gathered up together. Walk out freely. Try to get into a space and keep your eye on the steward.

The ponies will be called one by one into line. This may be a preliminary order but sometimes it is not at all and almost always your position can be changed by your individual performance. Some judges will ask for a set show giving you details of where they want you to trot on and canter and so on. If they do not the performance illustrated overleaf works well in most rings.

Walk out and stand in front of the judge. The judge will usually greet you with 'good morning/afternoon' and you should reply with same words. Even if you know the judge well you should make no other

Some native ponies can also compete in BSPS classes. This is Welsh Section A Aston Tinkerbell

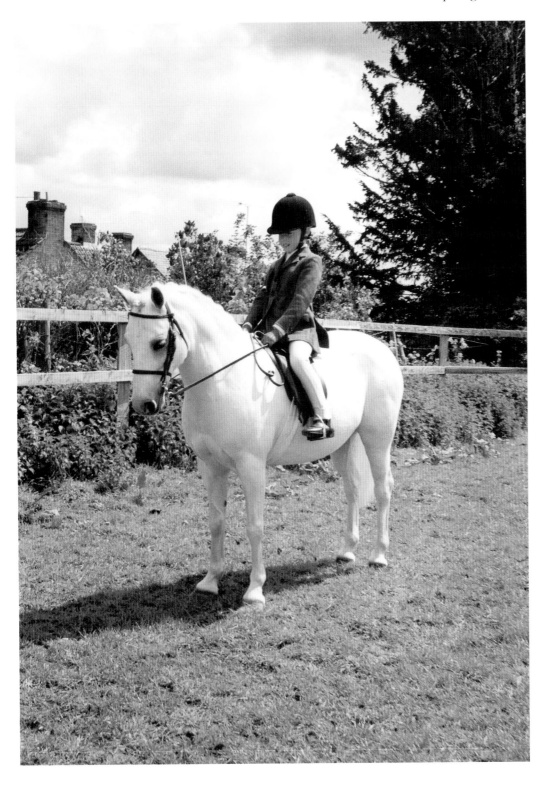

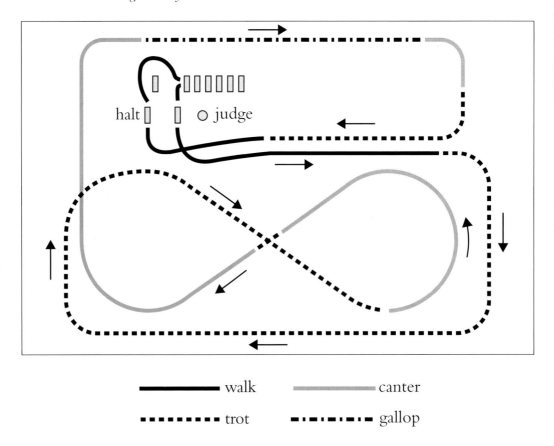

▬▬▬▬▬ walk	▬▬▬▬ canter
■·■·■·■·■ trot	■·■·■·■·■ gallop

Showing - individual performance

comment at all unless replying to a specific question such as 'how old is your pony?'. Stand your pony square, having him attentive but calm. If he is a fidget then you will have to keep your legs on him or play with the reins slightly or employ some other device to keep his attention. The judge will look round him and then send you off to do your show. Walk away from the judge and turn right onto the outside track. Proceed to trot, trotting along in front of the judge and all along the 'long side' of the ring. On reaching the corner go into canter, leading with the inside fore. Canter round in a half circle and as you get to the line of ponies, drop to trot. Trot across the diagonal, returning the canter on the other lead as you hit the outside track. Canter up the side, this time going behind the line of ponies. As you go along the back extend into gallop, returning to canter at the corner. Return to trot and then to walk as you go down the side of the ring, stopping where the judge can easily see you. You can drop your reins and salute by nodding your head or if you have any doubts about your pony standing still just salute by nodding your head and smiling.

This may complete the individual inspection or you may be required to come out again after all ridden shows have been completed. This second appearance will be in-hand. You should have an assistant ready at the ringside. They can come into the ring when the stewards have asked the ponies to strip. They should be very careful not to get in the way of competitors still doing their ridden show and they may bring a grooming kit with them. Your assistant will remove the pony's saddle, putting it on the ground behind him (but not too close!) He or she can then quickly brush away the saddle mark and do as much other tidying as the time will allow. If you are lucky enough to be first to go then you may well not have time for anything. When the steward signals to you, take your pony out of the line and stand him up in front of the judge. It is useful to have taught him the command to 'stand up' to get his attention. Throwing bits of grass about seems to be the fashion at present but it does not look very good from a judge's point of view. Keep him standing square and keep his attention. If he is really fidgety you can rustle a sweet paper in your pocket or tap your number behind your back with your cane. The judge may ask you how old the pony is but you should not volunteer any other information. It is especially bad form to take this as an opportunity to list the pony's previous successes.

When the judge gives you the signal walk away from her towards the side of the ring. It is not necessary to go very far – say walking for about ten seconds. Turn, pushing the pony away from you, so that you do not get between him and the judge. Go back towards the judge at trot, passing close to her and going on past her towards the end of the ring. You will turn right at

the ringside so that your track takes you round behind the line of ponies, where you drop to walk and return to your place in the line.

Your assistant will then re-saddle your pony and they will leave the ring, again being careful not to get in the way of other competitors. It should be said that some larger shows and championships have a dress code for grooms and may well require that your groom wears a hat. In any case they should be smartly and sensibly dressed and wearing stout shoes – for safety's sake if nothing else.

When everyone has shown their pony in-hand – or at least as many as the judge has asked to see and all the saddles are put on again, there will be a signal from the steward for a final walk round. Keep in the order that you were in line. Do not trot on unless the steward asks and do not get in closer and closer to the judge in ever decreasing circles.

The steward will call you in order to line up. Remember that it is not over until the rosettes have been given and sometimes a judge can still change their mind even at this late stage. You should have trained your pony at home to accept a rosette on his bridle. There have been several well-documented examples of ponies backing away or rearing when a rosette is offered and the judge having no alternative but to strip them of the championship. The prizewinners leave the ring at a canter on the right rein and the others leave directly towards the exit at a walk. The winner can do a second circuit of the ring at a gallop at larger shows or if asked to do so by the steward.

Championships

You may be lucky enough to be first or second in your class when there is a championship. It will tell you in the schedule whether there is a championship for your class or not. When the championship is called you go back into the ring with first and second prizewinners from various other sections. The procedure will be much the same as the original class. Ridden ponies may or may not do individual shows. They are not usually stripped again. The judge will choose a champion and reserve and may or may not line up all or some of the others. Anyone not lined up leaves the ring immediately at a walk.

Preparing for the show

Preparations for the show will have realistically started months or even years before. However, this section applies to the day before and the day of the show. If the weather is reasonably fine, you can bath your pony. See the section on coat care for full details. If it is winter or bad weather then you can give him a very thorough grooming or possibly a 'hot towel' wash. This involves a bucket of hand-hot water and an old towel or face flannel. The coat is rubbed thoroughly with the towelling, which is rinsed and wrung out at regular

Welsh Section D Joiners Southern Comfort is an accomplished competitor in Western riding events (here ridden by the author)

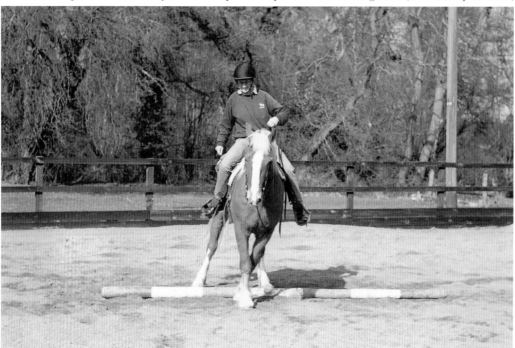

intervals. The amount of dirt that comes out this way is almost always very surprising!

It is always better if you can wash his mane and tail, no matter how cold or wet it is. Native manes and tails can look very unruly and by washing at least you can have an opportunity to flatten things down! The tail can be bandaged at the top and the rest put into three loose plaits and if it is a light colour thence into an old stocking. The mane can be plaited over to the right side after application of setting gel. The best kind of setting gel is that designed for humans and designated 'firm hold'. A hood can be useful to keep the mane flat if you do not want to plait for risk of too much curling. If your pony has white socks, it is usually best to wash them in the morning if you have time. If you wash the day before and put bandages on you risk flattening the feather too much. However, if you do have to wash the night before, get the bandages off in the morning and use thick foam travelling boots for the journey. They will offer the necessary protection to the legs without spoiling the effect of the feather too much.

In the hottest weather, do put a cotton summer sheet on even if you put nothing else on, if you have bathed the night before. Clean ponies are so very good at lying in dirt! No matter how clean the stable is when you go to bed he will still find something.

TACK

Tack must be cleaned and put ready in plenty of time. Put bridles together and check for small items such as lip straps and curb chains. Put the saddle together and make sure you have the stirrups, girth and any saddle pad or similar item. It is amazing how many girths are sold at shows to people who took it off to wash it and then forgot it! If you change your bit for different classes, remember to check this too.

GROOMING KIT

Everyone uses slightly different items in their grooming kit box; it can be useful to have a separate grooming kit for shows which stays in the lorry or tow vehicle at all times. Items, which may be forgotten, include fly repellent and sun block (for pink noses) in hot weather and tack cleaning equipment. Even though native ponies do not have plaits, a plaiting kit can be very useful for minor repairs and so on.

WATER

Do not rely on the show to have water available, even though many do. You will need enough water for the pony or ponies to drink and also for last minute washing and cleaning. Do not leave the water in containers from one show to the next. It will go stale and fussy ponies will not drink it.

FOOD

This means refreshments for you and for the pony. Obviously what you take is dependent on personal preference and on the length of time you will be away. Be warned though that the occasional show has no refreshment facilities at all and if you are unlucky you could end up very hungry.

PAPERWORK

The following items should be kept together in a file:

1. Vaccination certificates.
2. Height certificates.
3. Membership cards and pony registration or qualification cards.
4. Photocopies of your pony's registration certificates.
5. The schedule and/or catalogue for the current show. The numbers if you have been sent them and vehicle pass if it is needed.

You should also carry in your vehicle a very good road map and details of whatever breakdown organisation you belong to.

CLOTHES

Your riding or other showing clothes should be clean and put ready the day before the show. Do not forget boots, gloves, stick and other small items.

Good preparation for a show helps you to enjoy the day more. It is not always possible – or desirable – to buy or borrow forgotten items when you arrive without them. If you are very forgetful it may pay you to design your own checklist; run off several copies of the list on a computer or photocopier and religiously tick if off when preparing for every show.

Travelling

Most shows involve a journey either by lorry or by trailer. Travelling by lorry is always preferable except for very small ponies who do not seem to mind how they travel. Ponies get thrown about more in a trailer and will therefore have to expend more energy keeping their balance. A lorry is also invaluable for cups of tea in wet weather and for people to get changed in and so on. Many horse lorries can be driven without taking a special test. If you are in any doubt there should be a weight plate displayed on the lorry and the current weight restrictions can be obtained from your local Ministry of Transport office. For a trailer you will need a suitable towing vehicle and recent government legislation has limited the number of suitable vehicles. Again check with the Ministry of Transport rather than make a mistake. Anyone new to towing should have plenty of practise with an empty trailer before they venture out with their precious pony aboard.

Horses should be properly dressed for travelling. Rugs are not necessary and if they are used, should be put on tightly so that they cannot slip and upset the pony. The legs should be protected with boots or bandages, depending on personal preference and the tail protected from rubbing with a bandage or tail guard. Leather headcollars are always preferable for travelling because they will break in a major commotion such as an accident. A nylon headcollar is more likely to last longer than your pony's neck. In any case the pony should not be tied directly to the metal tie ring, but rather to a piece of doubled up bailer twine which is then attached to the ring. This will break more easily in the case of a problem.

Loading should have been practised well before the day of the show, but in case of

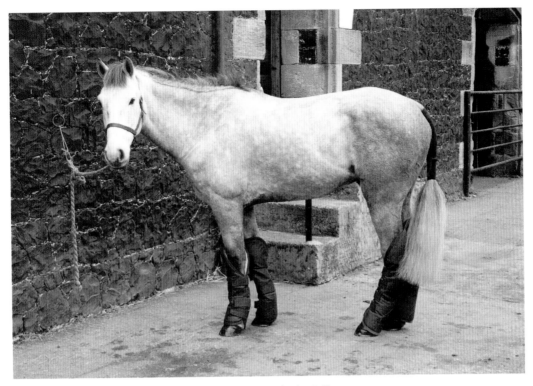

Prepared for a journey with travelling boots, tail bandage and leather headcollar

occasional problems, a lunge rein put behind the pony above the hocks and held at each end by a strong assistant usually changes ponies' minds about whether they want to load or not.

TRAVELLING TIPS

1. Leave in plenty of time! This cannot be stressed enough. When travelling on any journey with horses it will take you up to twice as long as it might in a car. If you are going to a venue that you have not been to before it might be more difficult to find than you think. If you are going to a county show the traffic might be re-routed from your planned route and there may be queues to get in.

2. Keep your lorry or towing vehicle and trailer in good order. Carry spare light bulbs. Make sure you belong to a breakdown organisation. There are organisations which offer cover especially designed for horse lorries and vehicles towing trailers. Choose one of these and keep your subscription up. As someone who was marooned in the wilds of Shropshire during a thunderstorm with three ponies and two worn out children, I guarantee the day will come when you were glad you did as I say and not as I do!

3. Check your route before you go. Check whether there are roadworks on your proposed route. AA Roadwatch is a service that you can telephone for this information.

At the show

Park where you are told to, but do leave plenty of room between yourself and the next vehicle. They might be wanting to tie up a large stallion to the side of their lorry. It is a matter of personal preference whether or not you tie up your pony outside or you leave him in the trailer or lorry. Your first job should be to go and get your numbers or enter if you need to and then go and find your ring and check on the progress of classes there.

Although most shows have loudspeaker announcements, you should not rely on them entirely. It is your responsibility to get yourself and your exhibit to the correct ring at the correct time. It is entirely a matter of personal preference whether you get the pony ready first and then ride him in or perhaps you would rather take your in-hand exhibit straight from the lorry into the ring so that he has extra sparkle. Whichever way works best for you is the right way to do it. Remember the main thing is to enjoy the day – you are doing this for fun after all!

The classes and criteria

IN-HAND

Youngstock – all youngstock – need to be good examples of their breed with good conformation and good straight action. If you have a second rate animal you may win on a day when entries are low but only the good ones win regularly – and no-one wins all the time. A colt should have a masculine look about him and a good helping of that

elusive quality known as presence. A filly can be less of a performer but should still be correct in every way.

RIDDEN CLASSES

Ridden ponies are judged both on their conformation of correctness of breed type and also on the way they perform under saddle. Manners are important, being more important the smaller the pony and rider combination gets. For example for a Welsh Cob stallion to be very free moving and onward going is correct (as long as he is not out of control!) If a Shetland pony with a seven or eight year old rider moves on too much appearing almost out of control the picture is very different and altogether less acceptable. A ridden pony should be obedient in all his paces and take the correct leg in canter. He should move in a correct outline, neither pulling (which often goes with overbending) nor coming above the bridle. In short he should look a pleasure to ride.

LEADING REIN AND FIRST RIDDEN

Only the smallest breeds compete in these classes, that is to say Shetland, Dartmoor, Exmoor, Welsh Section A and some Section B. An occasional New Forest might also be small enough for the height limit which is either 12hh or 12.2hh depending on which rules the show is held under. These ponies must go sweetly for their small rider, never pulling or going too fast. They must also go forward without too much encouragement, travelling along at all times at a sensible controlled pace. Obedience and manners are of paramount importance in these classes.

WORKING HUNTER PONY

The jumping round in these classes accounts for at least half of the allotted marks. Therefore it is essential that your pony jumps round without mistakes. He should travel at what is called a good hunting pace. This really means a working canter – a good strong canter without going too fast. He needs to jump fluently and neatly. As in every other class he should also be a good example of his breed with good conformation. However, if he is a moderate example of his breed but does jump very nicely then he will always win a few prizes along the way. The most beautiful pony will be nowhere if he does not jump.

STYLE AND PERFORMANCE

This is an increasingly popular version of a working hunter pony class. It starts in the same way with jumping round a course of rustic fences. The competitors are then required to execute what amounts to a short dressage test. This is set by the rules of whatever organisation it is held under. In these classes manners and obedience count far more than conformation and correctness.

Showing is all about enjoying your hobby and possibly winning a prize at the end of it all. You will never win much money even at the major championships. You will be exhausted, frustrated and disappointed but if you get home from the show and cannot wait for the next one then you are definitely hooked. If the pony that you take home with you is the one that *you* like best then who cares if he is first or last – you love him and that is all that matters!

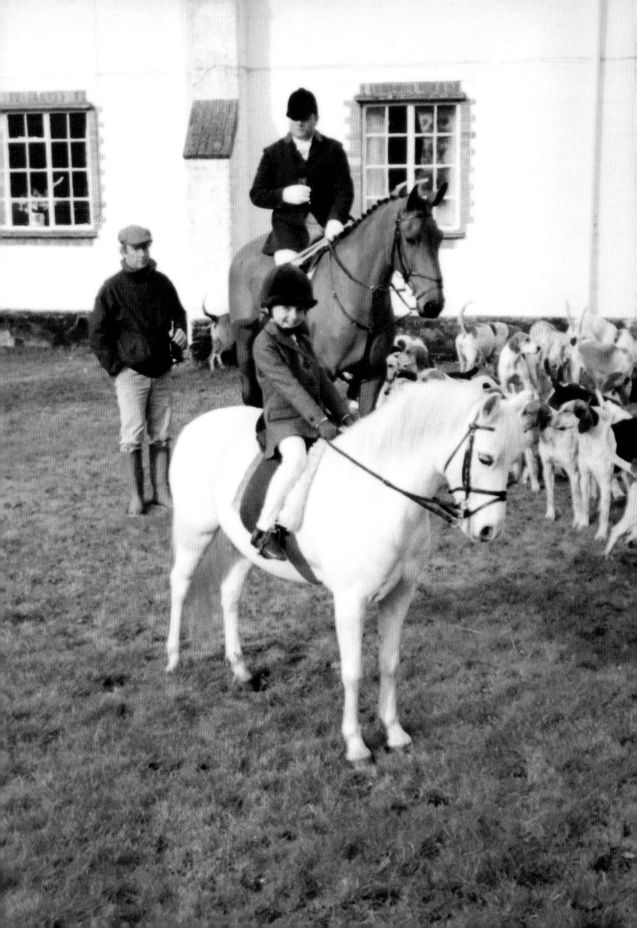

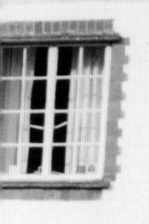

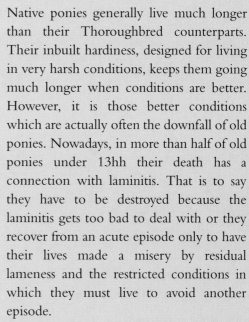

8

Sixteen Plus

Native ponies generally live much longer than their Thoroughbred counterparts. Their inbuilt hardiness, designed for living in very harsh conditions, keeps them going much longer when conditions are better. However, it is those better conditions which are actually often the downfall of old ponies. Nowadays, in more than half of old ponies under 13hh their death has a connection with laminitis. That is to say they have to be destroyed because the laminitis gets too bad to deal with or they recover from an acute episode only to have their lives made a misery by residual lameness and the restricted conditions in which they must live to avoid another episode.

Ponies can be expected to live easily into their twenties and a few make it into their thirties. Only very occasionally does a very resilient pony make forty. Some can be ridden right up to the end, but generally most retire by thirty and many by the time they reach twenty. Brood mares can have foals into their twenties but should not have a first foal after about the age of fourteen. You should take your veterinary

Aston Tinkerbell enjoying a day's hunting aged seventeen

surgeon's advice if you are contemplating a first foal for your teenage mare.

In general terms the older pony needs more care, will cost more to keep especially in the area of veterinary fees and you may well find yourself keeping him for up to twenty years without being able to use him. To sell a pony, which is aged more than about fifteen years, is not recommended. You have to be prepared to repay the pony for all that he has done for you. In any case a retired pony, grazing peacefully in the paddock is a great sight. You can look at him and remember all the good days and know that you are doing right by him.

Care

You must remember that your Dartmoor pony, if he lived wild at the turn of the century would not have lived a very long life. Many died as foals and even if he did grow up, he would not have lived more than about ten years. A pony with an injury or infection would either just have to curl up and die or if he recovered might well be impaired and die sooner than he would otherwise have done. Antibiotics and modern surgical practices have saved many ponies and kept them going for much longer than would be natural. However, this does not mean that you can neglect your pony and let nature take its course. Animal welfare standards today thankfully do not permit this to happen.

Your old pony needs a warm and comfortable stable. By their teenage years

many ponies have some arthritis and as those of you reading this who suffer the same condition will know, they need to be kept warm and dry. Whilst he can go out all day in reasonable weather, it might be useful to keep him in on the odd day which is very wet and windy. Cold, bright and windy weather is not usually a problem. If you have to put him out in wet weather a New Zealand rug can keep him dry even if he is not generally rugged up. Wet ponies standing in the stable at night soon get chilled.

If you have no stabling at all, then you can bed down a field shelter with plenty of straw or even put down straw in a sheltered corner of the field for him to lie down on. If he has to live out all the time you could use a New Zealand rug in December, January, February and March at least and you should have a spare one, so that you can change it each day and get it dry.

Teeth should be checked regularly. His food is a source of energy and thus warmth, so it is important that he can eat properly. If you notice that he is dropping half chewed food (known as 'quidding') then this is a sign that he has tooth problems. Other signs are bitting problems, rubbing his mouth on the fence and sometimes shaking the head.

Food should be best quality, especially hay. Most small ponies can live quite happily on good quality hay. By good quality, I do not mean the best seed hay, such as is given to racehorses! Good quality meadow hay, if it is well made and dust free is the most suitable type for ponies. Old ponies can have built up a hay dust allergy over the years and if this is the case, the hay must be soaked or steamed (see chapter 3). Haylage or other 'processed' hay is sometimes too rich for native ponies, especially when they get old. Older ponies who have worn down their teeth badly may not be able to cope with a haynet. Unless you really want to use a net, such as when travelling, most ponies are better fed on the floor. The exception to this is the pony who tramples in his food and then will not eat it.

There are special feeds designed for old ponies. They will contain a proper balance of vitamins and minerals and often various herbs thought to be useful for old ponies. They will give a very low protein feed in a tasty mixture and give interest to an otherwise boring diet especially for a pony whose grazing is restricted. However, overfeeding even of these low protein mixes will give problems to a laminitic pony. You should feed according to the instructions.

If you feed one of these complete mixes at the rate suggested by the manufacturer, you should not need to feed any other supplement. However, there are various supplements that are useful for certain conditions and you should refer to the 'health' section of this chapter for further details.

Carrots are nearly always relished by all ponies. Old ponies may have difficulty in chewing them and in this case they can be cut into long fingers to help. Never cut carrots into rings or other small pieces as these can cause a pony to choke. You can also grate carrot (a food processor can be very useful here) if your pony has very worn teeth.

If your old pony suffers from a decreasing appetite there are several measures you can try to help him feel more like eating. If you do not have much grass, you can pick him some long grass (or dandelions or sow thistles) if any is available from an uncontaminated source. Greenery from a roadside verge is not suitable, unless it is from a quiet lane.

A bran mash is very appetising especially in cold weather. Bran is not a good food source any more, because of the way that grain is processed nowadays. However, a properly made bran mash smells good enough to eat yourself and can be very tempting. See chapter 3 for a method of making a bran mash. Add a sprinkle of salt and some grated carrot and stir well. Other items that can be added include well-soaked sugar beet, or just the soaking water, drained off; honey; Guinness (about a teacup full) or linseed jelly.

The herb fenugreek is good for increasing appetite and for putting flesh on. This herb is usually purchased in powdered form, although you can try growing it in your garden to feed fresh for a really fussy feeder. A swede hung up on a short length of stout rope or placed in the manger, can encourage a pony to nibble. Never use a long length of rope in case he gets it round his neck.

My old ponies love baked bread. This is bread that has gone stale but not mouldy and which is baked in the oven until it is crisp. Whilst not being a strictly orthodox food it is obviously high in carbohydrate and (so the ponies say) utterly delicious.

Old age health problems

ARTHRITIS

The word means an inflammation of the joint. Arthritis can be the result of several different situations. Traumatic arthritis is the result of an injury. Rheumatoid arthritis is a degenerative condition. There are also various forms of arthritis caused by the animal being ill with a specific disease. In older horses and ponies the most common form is rheumatoid. The animal may have vague symptoms for months or even years before a definite lameness appears. At this stage crepitus, which is a grating sound, can sometimes be heard when the joint is flexed.

Diagnosis usually involves X-rays, although there are additional tests which can confirm the diagnosis. Treatment is with anti-inflammatory drugs which should always be prescribed by a veterinary surgeon after he has confirmed the diagnosis. The owner can do much in the way of supportive therapy to make the pony more comfortable.

Ensure as much as is possible that he is kept warm and dry. For arthritis in leg joints, woollen stable bandages put on overnight can be very comforting and supportive.

Bedding should be deep and banked up around the sides of the stable. Consideration should be given to using rubber matting under the bedding and on any areas not covered by bedding where the pony may stand.

Herbal remedies can be used alongside the conventional drugs to help with long term relief. Devil's claw is the most useful herb in these circumstances.

Veterinary advice concerning exercise should be followed to the letter. If the vet says half an hour walking and you start trotting on the roads and so on, you will make your pony's condition degenerate more rapidly, apart from causing him pain and suffering. When he is obviously hobbling around and/or when he starts to lose weight from pain, he should be put down to save him further suffering.

LAMINITIS

See chapter 4 for full information on this condition. In old age, a pony who is slightly lame may have chronic low level laminitis and this may be mistaken for arthritis. Since the treatment for these two conditions is different, you should always seek veterinary advice. (See also section on cancer below.)

CANCER

Old horses are prone to a number of cancers. A malignant tumour is a non-inflammatory, non-encapsulated new growth. They are normally difficult to define in extent and can metastasise into other areas of the body. Often when an old horse has a colic and has an operation, the cause of the colic is found to be tumours and huge growths weighing several pounds can be found inside the animal, without there being an external sign that there was a problem.

The form of cancer most likely to be actually seen by horse owners is that of melanoma. This is a black pigmented tumour, the tumour being coloured this way from melanin which is derived from

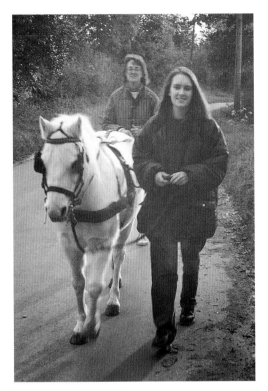

Learning a new skill aged nineteen

the colouring matter in hair and skin. They occur in horses which where originally grey and who have turned whiter with age. They are usually but not always malignant. Melanomas can come suddenly and stay very small for years only to increase just as suddenly without warning. They are of no bother unless they are in a position where tack or rugs might rub them. In this case care must be taken to avoid damage, as this can set off an increase in spread of the tumour. They also tend to bleed profusely when damaged.

One other form of cancer, which can be seen in old horses, is that of a 'rodent ulcer'. This can be caused by wearing boots which are too tight or not kept clean enough and for this reason is most often seen on the legs. It can also occur under a dirty headcollar left out in the field. It is a form not prone to metastasis but does destroy surface tissue and can become infected if not properly cared for.

HEART DISEASE

The most common heart problem in old horses is that of hypertrophy. This is an enlargement of the heart due to its being under constant strain, as in regular fast work or from a valvular problem or from high blood pressure. Whilst it is of no consequence in a younger horse, when the horse gets older and ceases work there is always a tendency for degenerative changes to occur. However, degeneration of the heart cannot be diagnosed with any certainty whilst the animal is alive. If your vet suspects that your pony may have heart problems there is not much you can do apart from giving him a quiet and uneventful life in retirement and ensuring that he stays under veterinary supervision. It is dangerous to ride any horse with heart problems – he may drop down dead whilst you are on his back. Having actually seen this happen and seen the rider dreadfully injured, I would urge you to follow your vet's advice to the letter.

Retirement

Many ponies – especially native ponies – have many years of happy retirement or semi-retirement. This should definitely not mean being stuck in a field and visited on high days and holidays. As has already been said old ponies need *more* care than younger ones. They often relish human company having had years of regular riding. They love routine and know better than you what comes next in the daily pattern. Aston Tinkerbell is now well over twenty. Each morning when I let her out she goes immediately to the feed shed and waits for me to get her morning feed. If I go to fill water buckets first or do some other jobs, she comes steaming after me shaking her head and making sure I know in no uncertain terms that feed comes first! This kind of behaviour makes old ponies an absolute delight around the yard.

So, when should you retire your pony? Obviously some mares retire from a ridden career to have children. If a brood mare has not got in foal for three years running or two years if she has had previous foals and is over fifteen years old, retirement might be on the cards. If your ridden pony develops a condition which means riding causes him pain, he should be retired. Otherwise you should take veterinary advice on what kind of work, if any, he is up to doing at any stage. Some ponies, whilst not being able to have a full-time ridden job can very happily manage the occasional slow ride or can become very useful to Riding for the Disabled. Many groups use ponies owned by private owners who take them along each week to give great pleasure to disabled riders without causing the pony any great exertion. Some ponies take on a very useful role in retirement in looking after youngstock. Youngsters can learn a great deal from being around an older and wiser pony.

The end

How will you know your old pony cannot go on any longer? It may of course happen that he develops an acute problem which because of his age and infirmity is impossible to treat. You may decide that a long-standing illness cannot go on any longer. You may just find him one morning in his stable or field. The most difficult of these three scenarios is the middle one. You are in effect playing God with the life of your animal. If you have had him for many years it is all too easy to prolong the decision and tell yourself that whilst he can still hobble about he is happy – but is he? At what point are you keeping this animal alive purely for selfish reasons? He has been a good servant to you for however many years you have had him and whilst you could not imagine life without him, you really owe it to him to prevent him from suffering. Remember – animals know nothing at all about tomorrow. They do not look forward to events or happenings. They live only in the moment and in that moment if they are feeling pain and discomfort that is all they know. They cannot think 'Perhaps my owner will give me some medicine tomorrow and I will feel better'. They cannot think 'I hope I hang on long enough to go back in the big field in the summer'. They only know *now*.

So how do you make the decision? Start by getting your veterinary surgeon involved. Most vets will not put down a pony unless they think it is necessary. It can be quite useful to take a photograph of your old pony every couple of months or so. When you see him every day, you will not notice gradual deterioration too readily. When you look at the photo from two months before and then perhaps four months before, you will be able to see the change for yourself and that may help you make up your mind. If he cannot trot when you put him out; if he cannot get up and lie down relatively easily; if he stops eating and his teeth are in good order; if his coat goes dull, staring and patchy or he groans when moving about, he is probably nearing or at the end. If he has to be on a maximum dose of painkiller for more than three months you should also review the situation.

When you have made the final decision, book the vet not more than twenty-four hours ahead. This will make it easier for you. Give the pony some Bach Flowers Rescue Remedy every half-hour on the day and take the same dose yourself. You will have to discuss with the vet beforehand whether he is to shoot the pony or use a lethal injection. There is for and against for both methods. Shooting is quick and almost always the pony drops without knowing what has happened. For some owners, however, it seems very brutal. They cannot bear the thought of inflicting a wound. Other horses should be moved away from the scene because they can become very distressed.

An injection can also have an immediate effect, especially if the pony is very old and has a weak heart. However, for a pony which might have bad arthritis but has a strong constitution otherwise, one injection might not be enough and whilst he may drop down immediately, he could take up to ten minutes or more to die. This

can be distressing for the owner and in the rare case where the pony tries to get up again can be distressing for the pony too. Even the very best vet can get caught out occasionally.

The next problem is the body. You can arrange for the local hunt to collect the body if he has been shot (hunts cannot accept ponies killed by lethal injection) but many areas have no hunting nearby and this might not therefore be feasible. You can arrange to bury him on your own land. There are by-laws governing such matters together with regulations about the depth of the hole and so on. You must consult your local council well in advance (unless this is impossible because the death is sudden). You will need to hire a digger (unless you happen to have one) and this too should be booked in advance if possible. You can have your pony cremated, so that you can scatter his ashes on his favourite paddock. Many abattoirs now have incineration facilities, because of the need to dispose of BSE-infected cattle. They will clean out the incinerator and do a special running of the furnace just for your pony if you pay an appropriate fee. There are crematoriums specialising in pet cremations. They will cremate your pet and give you the ashes in a casket or scatter them on their garden of remembrance. This is, however, very expensive, the cost running into hundreds of pounds.

The most usual method of disposal is for your local slaughterhouse to collect the body. Some companies will shoot the pony too if you want this. Whilst sentiment is an issue for most people, you might like to think that the body is in fact just his old clothes. The real pony – his soul if you like to call it that – will always be there. You will always have your memories; the photographs; the video and possibly the rosettes and cups. If you do right by your animals whilst they are alive

that is all that you can do for them.

You might like to think about donating a trophy to a show in memory of your pony or making a donation to a charity such as Riding for the Disabled to make a permanent reminder.

Useful Addresses

British Association for Homoeopathic
Veterinary Surgeons,
Chinham House, Stanford in the Vale,
Nr. Faringdon, Oxfordshire, SN7 8NQ
Tel: 01367 710324

The British Horse Society,
Stoneleigh Deer Park, Kenilworth,
Warwickshire, CV8 2XZ
Tel: 01926 707700
Fax: 01926 707800
e-mail: enquiry@bhs.org.uk
Web site: www.bhs.org.uk

British Show Pony Society,
124 Green End Road, Sawtry,
Huntingdon, Cambridgeshire,
PE17 5XA
Tel: 01487 831376

Dales Pony Society,
Greystones, Glebe Avenue,
Great Longstone, Bakewell, Derbyshire,
DE45 1TY
Tel: 01629 640439

Dartmoor Pony Society,
57 Pykes Down, Ivybridge, Devon,
PL21 0BY
Tel: 01752 987053

English Connemara Society,
Woodland St Mary Cottage,
Woodland St Mary, Lambourn, Berkshire,
RG1 7SL
Tel: 01488 73313

Exmoor Pony Society,
Glenfern, Waddicombe, Dulverton,
Somerset, TA22 9RY
Tel: 01398 341490

Farriers Registration Council,
Sefton House, Adam Court, Newark
Road, Peterborough, PE1 5PP
Tel: 01733 319911

Fell Pony Society,
Keepers Cottage, Guyzance, Acklington,
Northumberland, NE65 9AA
Tel: 01670 761117

Highland Pony Society,
22 York Place, Perth, PH2 8EH
Tel: 01738 451861

National Foaling Bank,
Meretown Stud, Meretown, Nr. Newport,
Shropshire
Tel: 01952 811234

National Pony Society,
Willingdon House, 102 High Street,
Alton, Hampshire, GU34 1EN
Tel: 01420 88333

New Forest Pony and Cattle Breeding
Society,
Beacon Cottage, Burley, Ringwood,
Hampshire, NH24 4EW
Tel: 01425 402272

Ponies UK,
Chesham House,
56 Green End Road, Sawtry,
Huntingdon, Cambridgeshire,
PE17 5UY
Tel: 01487 830278

Shetland Pony Stud Book Society,
Shetland House,
 22 York Place, Perth,
PH2 8EH
Tel: 01738 623471

Welsh Pony and Cob Society,
6 Chalybeate Street, Aberystwyth,
Caredigion, SY23 1HS
Tel: 01970 617501

Further Reading

ABC of Horse and Pony Problems, Josephine Knowles, J. A. Allen

Allen Book of Ponies, Carolyn Henderson and Jennifer Bell, J. A. Allen

Allen Photographic Guides, J. A. Allen

Horse and Stable Management, Jeremy Houghton Brown and Vincent Powell-Smith, BSP

Horse Nutrition and Feeding, Sarah Pilliner, BSP

Pasture Management for Horses and Ponies, Gillian McCarthy, BSP

Practical Horse and Pony Nutrition, Gillian McCarthy, J. A. Allen

Showing Native Ponies, Jenny Morgan, Kenilworth Press

Showing the Ridden Pony, Caroline Akrill, J. A. Allen

The Allen Equine Dictionary, Maria Belknap, J. A. Allen

The BHS Complete Manual of Stable Management, Kenilworth Press

The Shetland Pony, Anna Hodson, J. A. Allen

The Welsh Cob, Dr Wynne Davies J. A. Allen

Threshold Picture Guides Series, Kenilworth Press

Veterinary Care of the Horse, Sue Devereux, J. A. Allen

Welsh Mountain Pony, Dr Wynne Davies J. A. Allen

Welsh Ponies and Cobs, Dr Wynne Davies J. A. Allen

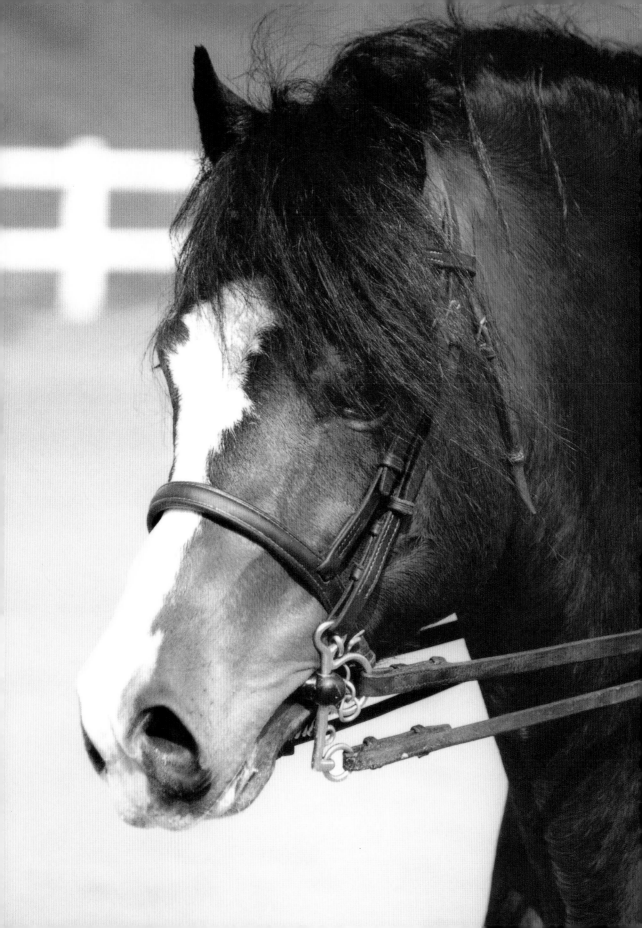

Index

Index